Title: NCLEX RN CASE STUDIES EXAM PRACTICE BOOTCAMP

Author: Anita Bhattarai
ISBN: 9798877742420
Imprint: Independently published
Copyright © 2024 Anita Bhattarai
Cover design by Gunjan Subedi

All rights reserved. No part of this book may be reproduced or transmitted in any form or by any means, electronic or mechanical, including photocopying, recording, or any information storage and retrieval system, without permission in writing from the author, except for brief quotations in critical articles or reviews.

Disclaimer: This book, "NCLEX RN CASE STUDIES EXAM PRACTICE BOOTCAMP," is intended to provide comprehensive information and strategies for nurses preparing for the NCLEX RN exam. While every effort has been made to ensure the accuracy and effectiveness of the content within, it is important to note the following:

Not a Replacement for Professional Advice: This book is not a substitute for professional medical or nursing advice, interventions, or treatment. It is intended solely as a study aid and reference guide to assist in NCLEX RN exam preparation.

Individual Responsibility: Readers are responsible for their own actions and decisions based on the information provided in this book. The author and publisher do not accept responsibility for any consequences resulting from actions taken by readers in relation to the content presented.

Variability in Exam Performance: Passing the NCLEX RN exam requires a combination of knowledge, critical thinking, and test-taking skills. While this book offers valuable resources, it cannot guarantee success on the NCLEX RN exam, as individual performance may vary.

Additional Study Materials (continued): While this book provides a comprehensive guide to NCLEX RN exam preparation, candidates are encouraged to diversify their study resources. Utilize a wide range of supplementary materials, such as official NCLEX RN study guides, practice exams, and educational courses, to ensure a well-rounded and thorough review of the exam content.

The terms 'NCLEX RN' and 'NCSBN' (National Council of State Boards of Nursing) are not my proprietary. It is important to note that passing the NCLEX RN exam requires a combination of knowledge, critical thinking, and test-taking skills. While this book may provide helpful resources, it is not a guarantee of passing the NCLEX RN exam, and it is recommended to utilize a variety of study materials and resources to prepare adequately.

First Printing: 2024

Dedication

Dedicated to all the busy nurses and nursing students, valiantly navigating the intricate dance of work, home, and family commitments. You, the unsung heroes, epitomize dedication, working tirelessly to deliver exceptional care while managing an array of responsibilities at home. Your unwavering commitment to both profession and family serves as a profound inspiration.

Understanding the unique struggles you face, I acknowledge the immense difficulty of balancing these multifaceted roles. Yet, amidst it all, you possess the audacity to dream big and pursue your goals. Your strength, perseverance, and determination embody the true spirit of nursing, and I am genuinely awestruck by your resolute character.

To every busy nurse reading these lines, remember you are not alone. With over a decade in this profession, I've witnessed your struggles and triumphs. I see you, I commend you, and I express heartfelt gratitude for your invaluable service to the nursing community. This book is dedicated to you, recognizing your challenges and designed to provide support, especially through the inclusion of crucial case studies. May it serve as a guiding light, helping you navigate the complexities of your professional journey with confidence and success.

ACKNOWLEDGEMENT

Writing a book is not a solo effort, and this one is no exception. Though I am the author, this book is the result of a collective approach of many circumstances and the motivation from many people.

First and foremost, I would like to express my heartfelt gratitude to all the nurses who work tirelessly to provide excellent care to patients. Your dedication and commitment inspire me every day.

I also want to thank my family and friends who supported me throughout this journey. Many friends like me know how challenging it is to balance work and family responsibilities. Therefore, I am particularly thankful to my husband, my better half, Gunjan Subedi, who supported me in everything, from preparing dinner to taking care of our child, so that I could focus on writing this book. Thank you for coffee, thank you for support, thank you for encouragement.

Furthermore, I want to express my gratitude to all the students who have inspired me to be a helpful teacher. Your success looks like my own victory, and I am honored to be part of your learning journey.

Finally, I would like to thank my parents for their unwavering love and support throughout my life. Their encouragement and guidance have been instrumental in shaping who I am today.

Once again, thank you to all the wonderful people who have contributed to the creation of this book.

-Anita Bhattarai

Table of Contents

Table of Contents 4

Feeling Lucky ? 5

Case Study Question : Introduction 6

Effective Strategies for Approaching Case Studies 8

Case Study Questions Presentation Style 9

Some key notes for exam 11

Other types of Questions 14

CASE STUDY 1 : Clinical Presentation of Parkinson's Disease 33

CASE STUDY 2: Early Diagnosis and Management of Type 2 Diabetes Mellitus. 39

CASE STUDY 3: Challenges and Management of Prolonged Labor in Primigravida 44

CASE STUDY 4: Management Strategies for Paranoid Schizophrenia 50

CASE STUDY 5: Effective Transfusion Management 58

CASE STUDY 6: Management of Electrolyte Imbalance 63

CASE STUDY 7: Management of Acute Exacerbation of Asthma 67

CASE STUDY 8: Management and Treatment Strategies for Burn Injuries 71

CASE STUDY 9: Managing Epilepsy 75

CASE STUDY 10: Prevention and Management Strategies for Pressure Ulcers 80

CASE STUDY 11: Management Approaches for Rheumatoid Arthritis 84

CASE STUDY 12: Diagnosis and Management of Adrenal Insufficiency 88

CASE STUDY 13: Hypothyroidism Diagnosis and Management 93

CASE STUDY 14 : Diagnosis and Management of Type 2 Diabetes Mellitus 98

CASE STUDY 15: Anxiety Disorders and Cardiovascular Health 104

Case Study 16: Management of Geriatric Patients 109

CASE STUDY 17: Infection Control in a Postoperative Patient 115

CASE STUDY 18 : Nutrition and Medication Interaction 121

Bibliography 128

Feeling Lucky ?

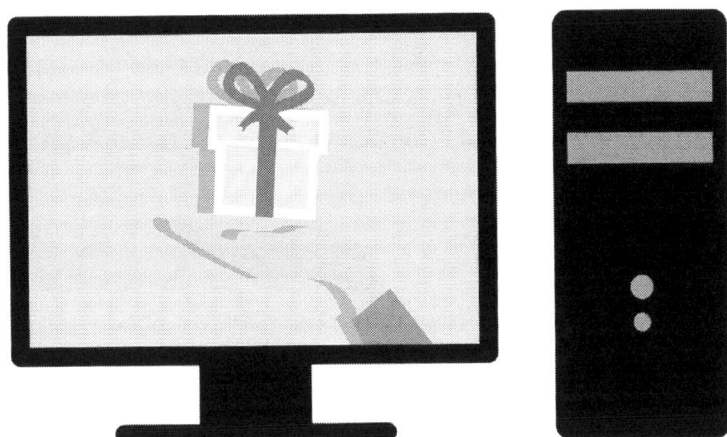

Attention all nursing students!

Every month, we randomly select 100 students to participate in our free fast track NCLEX RN practice course. This could be your chance to join and take the first step towards achieving your dream of becoming a registered nurse. Our course is tailored to provide you with comprehensive and effective practice resources that will help you build the necessary knowledge and skills to excel in your exam. Our expertly crafted study materials and practice tests will set you on the path to success. Don't miss out on this opportunity, sign up now and start your journey to becoming a registered nurse!

LINK- www.nclexmentors.com/freenclexcrashcourse

For other free resources, join us,

Youtube: https://www.youtube.com/@nextgenerationnclexmentors

Facebook (New Page):
https://www.facebook.com/groups/2295458660638596

Case Study Question : Introduction

The structure of questions in the Next Generation NCLEX (NGN) maintains some similarities with the previous format but introduces additional case study questions and standalone questions. These modifications aim to evaluate candidates' clinical judgment and decision-making skills in a more thorough and pragmatic manner.

A noteworthy aspect of the NGN exam is the incorporation of case study questions designed to assess a candidate's application of critical thinking in real-life patient scenarios. Each case study comprises six questions related to the presented scenario, encompassing the patient's health history/nurse notes, vital signs, lab values, and medications.

The case study questions are displayed on the right side of the screen, accompanied by multiple options for selection. As candidates answer each question, the subsequent query appears on the right side, linked to the same case study. These six questions, associated with each case study, evaluate various cognitive skills:

Recognition of cues
Analysis of cues
Prioritization of hypotheses
Generation of solutions
Taking appropriate action
Evaluation of outcomes

What do these cognitive skills mean?

Recognition of Cues:

The ability to identify relevant information or cues from a given scenario or case study.
Example: In a patient case study, recognizing signs and symptoms such as increased heart rate, shortness of breath, and chest pain as potential cues for a cardiovascular issue.

Analysis of Cues:

The skill of examining and interpreting the identified cues to understand their significance and implications.
Example: After recognizing the cues mentioned above, analyzing them to understand that they might indicate a possible myocardial infarction or heart attack.

Prioritization of Hypotheses:

The ability to rank or prioritize potential explanations or hypotheses based on the analysis of cues.
Example: Considering various hypotheses for the patient's symptoms, prioritizing the possibility of a heart attack over other potential causes like anxiety or indigestion.

Generation of Solutions:

Creating and proposing potential actions or solutions based on the prioritized hypotheses.

Example: If a heart attack is considered a high-priority hypothesis, generating solutions could involve immediate interventions such as administering aspirin, calling for emergency medical assistance, and preparing for possible cardiac interventions.

Taking Appropriate Action:

Implementing the chosen solution or intervention based on the prioritized hypotheses.
Example: Taking appropriate action involves actually calling for emergency medical assistance, administering aspirin, and preparing the patient for transportation to a healthcare facility for further evaluation and treatment.

Evaluation of Outcomes:

Assessing the results or outcomes of the actions taken to determine their effectiveness and any subsequent steps needed.
Example: After the patient has received medical attention, evaluating outcomes involves assessing whether the interventions had a positive effect on the patient's condition, monitoring for any complications, and adjusting the care plan as necessary.

To succeed in the NGN exam, candidates should adopt a systematic approach to tackle case study questions. This involves a meticulous review of the case study information, identification of relevant cues, analysis to generate a prioritized list of hypotheses, development of solutions based on hypotheses, taking appropriate action, and evaluating outcomes.

For instance, in a case study where a patient presents with severe abdominal pain, the candidate must identify pertinent cues such as vital signs, medical history, and medications. Analyzing these cues may lead to hypotheses like appendicitis or gastroenteritis. Subsequently, the candidate devises a plan, evaluates its effectiveness based on the patient's response, and adjusts the approach as needed.

Effective Strategies for Approaching Case Studies

Next-generation NCLEX-RN case study questions require a multifaceted approach for effective handling. Here's a detailed breakdown of the strategies outlined:

Comprehensive Reading:

Before attempting to answer any questions, thoroughly read the entire case study to establish a solid foundation. This includes delving into the patient's medical history, symptoms, and vital signs.
Example: If the case study involves a patient presenting with chest pain, make sure to understand the duration, characteristics of pain, associated symptoms, and any relevant past medical history like heart disease or diabetes.

Problem Identification:

Pinpoint the primary issue or medical condition affecting the patient. This step is crucial for prioritizing interventions and ensuring that the most critical aspects are addressed promptly.
Example: In a case study depicting a patient with shortness of breath, identifying whether the primary problem is respiratory, cardiac, or related to other factors helps in formulating appropriate interventions.

Nursing Knowledge Application:

Apply your nursing knowledge to connect the dots between symptoms, potential causes, and underlying factors. This involves drawing on your understanding of anatomy, physiology, and pathophysiology.
Example: If a case study involves a patient with altered mental status, use your nursing knowledge to explore potential causes such as hypoxia, metabolic disturbances, or neurological issues.

Multiple Perspectives:

Look at the case study from various angles, including the patient's perspective, the healthcare team's standpoint, and ethical or legal considerations. This broadens your understanding of the scenario and enhances critical thinking.
Example: Consider a case where a patient refuses a prescribed treatment. Explore the situation from the patient's autonomy, the healthcare team's duty to provide optimal care, and any legal or ethical implications surrounding informed consent.

Plan of Care Development:

Based on the identified problem and related issues, formulate a comprehensive plan of care. Prioritize evidence-based interventions that align with the patient's needs and the healthcare context.
Example: If the case study involves a patient with diabetes and a foot ulcer, develop a plan addressing wound care, glycemic control, patient education, and collaboration with other healthcare professionals.

Case Study Questions Presentation Style

The NCLEX-RN case study questions are presented in a split-screen format, designed to provide a comprehensive scenario for candidates to analyze. The screen is divided into two main sections: the left-hand side and the right-hand side.

Left-hand Side:

Patient Information: The left side typically contains essential patient information, including demographics, medical history, current symptoms, and any relevant diagnostic data. This information sets the stage for the case study scenario and provides context for the questions that follow.

Vital Signs and Lab Results: Important vital signs, laboratory results, and diagnostic findings pertinent to the case are often displayed on the left side. Candidates must pay close attention to these details as they can impact the decision-making process.

Medication List: A list of medications the patient is currently taking or has been prescribed may be included. Understanding the patient's medication regimen is crucial for making informed clinical judgments.

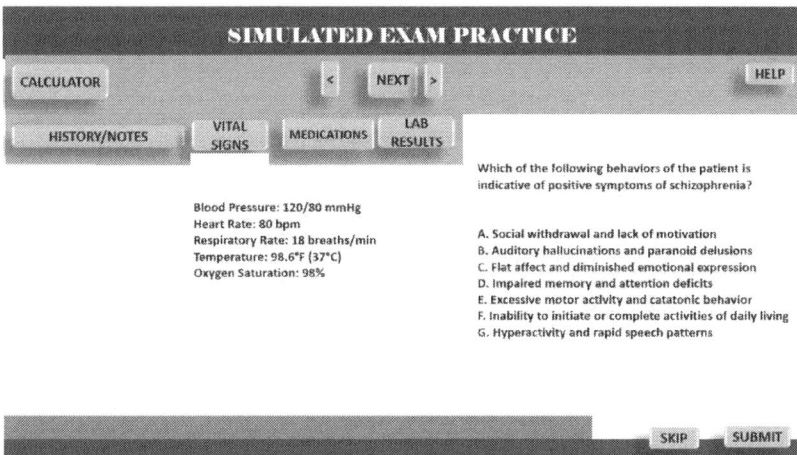

Source to video: https://www.youtube.com/@nextgenerationnclexmentors

Right-hand Side:

Case Study Questions: The right side of the screen presents the actual case study questions. These questions may include multiple-choice, select-all-that-apply (SATA), or other question types. Candidates must use the information provided on the left side to answer these questions accurately.

Decision Tree or Flowchart: Some case study questions may feature a decision tree or flowchart on the right side, guiding candidates through a step-by-step process in their decision-making. This visual aid helps organize thoughts and responses logically.

Patient Responses: As candidates progress through the case study, the right side may dynamically update to display patient responses to interventions or changes in condition. This feature allows candidates to assess the effectiveness of their decisions in real-time.

Tips for Approaching Case Study Questions:

Read Carefully: Take the time to thoroughly read and understand the patient information, vital signs, and other details provided on the left side before attempting to answer questions.

Analyze Patient Responses: Monitor how the patient's condition evolves as you answer each question. Adjust your approach based on the outcomes presented on the right side of the screen.

Use the Decision Tree: If available, leverage decision trees or flowcharts to systematically approach the case study questions. These tools can help organize your thought process.

Prioritize Interventions: Identify the most urgent interventions based on the patient's condition and prioritize them when answering questions. This mirrors real-world clinical decision-making.

Some Key Notes for Exam

Number of Case Study Questions: All exam writers will see three scored case studies, and each case study is composed of six items, for a total of 18 items.

Scoring System: The Next Generation NCLEX introduces a new scoring methodology known as polytomous (partial credit) scoring4. The scoring system for the Next Generation NCLEX exam will be based on one of three methods56:

0/1 Scoring: You earn one point for selecting the correct answer and zero points for an incorrect answer.
+/- Scoring: Awards points for correct selections and subtracts points for incorrect selections7.
Rationale Scoring: Earn points when both responses in the pair are correct8.
Difficulty Level: The Next Generation NCLEX is expected to be more challenging as it contains more in-depth questions and real-life scenarios9. However, it's designed to better measure a student's clinical judgment, so it's not impossible to pass104.

Consequences of Answering Incorrectly: In the new NGN-style questions, partial credit is now given in three different ways: ± scoring, Dyad scoring, and Triad scoring7. For example, in +/- scoring, you earn one point for each correct response, but lose one point for each incorrect response47.

Time Management: Candidates will still have up to five hours to complete the NCLEX-RN or NCLEX-PN exam. The items are presented in sequential order, so candidates progress through all six steps of the NCSBN Clinical Judgment Measurement Model (NCJMM), which includes recognizing cues, analyzing cues, prioritizing hypotheses, generating solutions, taking actions, and evaluating outcomes

For example, let's consider the following case study:

Patient's History: Madan, a 45-year-old male, was admitted to the hospital with a history of severe bleeding from an injury. He was diagnosed with a severe case of thrombocytopenia and was in need of an immediate blood transfusion.
end of strategy

Nurse's Notes:
• Assessed the patient's identification band and matched it with the name on the blood sample
• Checked the Rh and ABO compatibility of the blood sample before transfusing
• Transfused 1 unit of packed red blood cells to increase the erythrocytes for oxygen transportation
• Transfused 2 units of platelets to address the thrombocytopenia and improve clotting
• Monitored the patient's vital signs during and after the transfusion
• Checked the laboratory values for erythrocyte and platelet count after 4-6 hours of transfusion

Vital Signs:

Temperature 98.8°F- Normal- 98.6°F (37°C)
Heart rate (pulse): 75 bpm. Normal-60 to 100 beats per minute
Respiratory rate: 15 beats per minute. Normal range is 12 to 20 breaths per minute
Blood pressure: 118/80

Physician's Order:
• Transfuse 1 unit of packed red blood cells
• Transfuse 2 units of platelets
• Check laboratory values for erythrocyte and platelet count after 4-6 hours
• Monitor vital signs during and after transfusion

Lab Values:
• Hemoglobin increased from 8 g/dL to 9 g/dL after transfusion
• Hematocrit increased from 24% to 27% after transfusion
• Platelet count increased from 50,000 to 150,000 after transfusion

Which of the following is a primary concern for Madan as noted in the case study?

A. Increased hemoglobin levels
B. Rh and ABO compatibility of the blood sample
C. Thrombocytopenia
D. Increased hematocrit levels

Answer: C. Thrombocytopenia

Strategy description: To effectively approach a case study, a comprehensive reading of the case study is essential to gain a thorough understanding of the patient's medical history, symptoms, vital signs, and any other relevant information. Once you have read the case study, identify the primary problem or concern that the patient is facing. This will help you prioritize your interventions and focus your attention on the most critical issues. In this case, the primary concern is Madan's thrombocytopenia as evidenced by the physician's order and nurse's notes regarding the transfusion of platelets. Checking the laboratory values after the transfusion helps to monitor the effectiveness of the intervention.

Another Example:

Patient's History: A 65-year-old male patient has been admitted with symptoms of shortness of breath, cough, and wheezing. He has a history of smoking and asthma.

Nurse's Notes:
- Observed shortness of breath and wheezing while breathing
- Chest sounds congested with wheezing and crackles
- Pulse rate elevated at 120 bpm, Blood pressure is 90/60 mmHg
- Oxygen saturation is recorded at 88% on room air

Physician's Order:
- ABG test to evaluate acid-base balance
- Chest X-ray to evaluate lung condition
- Spirometry to evaluate lung function
- Nebulization to relieve wheezing and shortness of breath
- Bronchodilators to open up airways

Lab Values: ABG test results:
- pH: 7.25
- PaCO2: 50 mm Hg
- HCO3: 20 mEq/L
- O2 Sat: 88%

Which of the following interventions is most likely to be included in the plan of care for a patient with shortness of breath, wheezing, and an ABG result showing a low pH and high PaCO2 levels?

A) Administer pain medication
B) Schedule an appointment with a physical therapist
C) Administer a nebulization treatment
D) Order a chest X-ray

Strategy: The question requires applying the strategy of problem identification by identifying the primary problem, which is shortness of breath and wheezing. Then, utilizing nursing knowledge and expertise to identify the potential causes and generating a comprehensive understanding of the patient's condition by reviewing the nurse's notes, physician's orders, and lab values. Finally, selecting the appropriate intervention based on the provided information.

Answer: C) Administer a nebulization treatment, as it is the most appropriate intervention for a patient with shortness of breath and wheezing. The ABG result indicating a low pH and high PaCO2 levels suggest respiratory acidosis, which can be treated with bronchodilators such as nebulization to relieve wheezing and open up airways, improving oxygenation and reducing CO2 retention. Option A, administering pain medication, is not relevant to the patient's current condition. Option B, scheduling an appointment with a physical therapist, is not an immediate intervention for the patient's acute symptoms. Option D, ordering a chest X-ray, may be helpful in evaluating lung condition, but it is not the most appropriate intervention for addressing the patient's immediate respiratory distress.

Other types of Questions

1. **Extended Multiple Options or Multiple Response Questions**

One of the key features that this exam shares with its predecessor is the utilization of multiple-choice questions, which can include either multiple options or multiple answers for a single question. These types of questions provide candidates with a list of choices, and they must select the correct answer from that list.

In this exam, the multiple-choice questions can also be extended, meaning that there may be many more options to choose from. This could require candidates to take a more comprehensive approach to answer the question, as they must carefully consider each option before selecting the correct one.

It is worth noting that this exam has a partial marking system for multiple-response questions. This means that candidates will receive marks for each correct option selected, rather than the previous system where they would receive zero marks if even one option was incorrect. For example, if a question has four possible answers and the candidate selects two correct options and two incorrect options, they will receive partial credit for the two correct options selected.

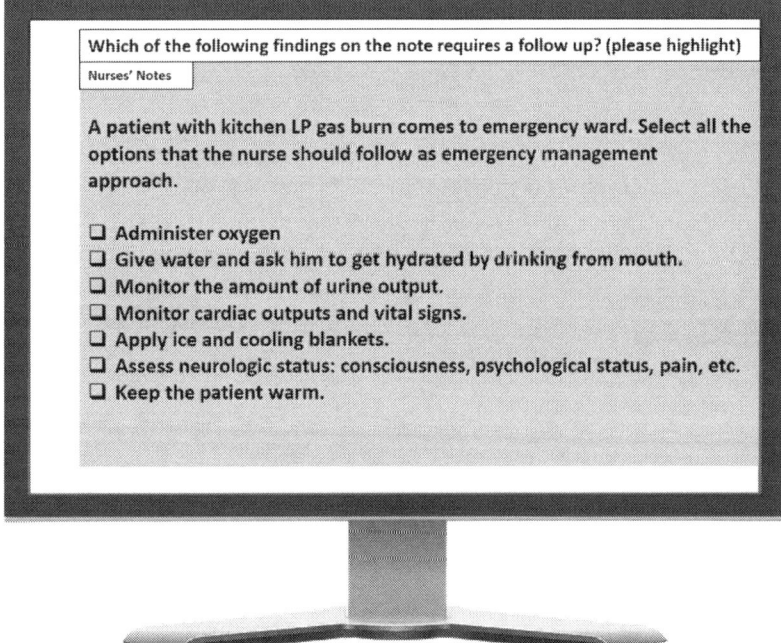
113

Strategies for extended multiple answers questions:
The Multiple Answer Case Study questions in the Next Gen NCLEX exam require you to identify all the correct answers to a particular scenario or problem. To effectively solve such questions, you can follow these step-by-step approaches:

1. **Understand the scenario and question:**

Read the case study scenario carefully, identify the key issues, and determine the type of question being asked. It is important to understand the context and what is being asked of you to choose the correct answers.

Example:

A case study scenario might describe a patient with heart failure who is prescribed multiple medications, and the question might ask which medications should be withheld if the patient has a low blood pressure reading.

2. **Identify possible answers:**

After understanding the scenario and question, generate a list of possible answers by reviewing your knowledge and the given information. It is essential to review all options before selecting the correct answers.

Example:

In the heart failure case study scenario, possible answers might include all the medications the patient is taking, as well as additional medications that could potentially affect blood pressure.

3. **Eliminate incorrect answers:**

Review each option and eliminate those that are not relevant or do not apply to the scenario. Consider the context of the scenario and the question being asked. This step helps to narrow down your options and select the correct answers.

Example:

In the heart failure case study scenario, medications that do not affect blood pressure or have no direct effect on heart failure management could be eliminated as incorrect answers.

4. **Select the correct answers:**

After eliminating incorrect answers, identify the correct answers by choosing the options that directly apply to the scenario and the question being asked. Review your choices and ensure that you have selected all the correct options.

Example:

In the heart failure case study scenario, the correct answers might include medications that lower blood pressure, such as diuretics and ACE inhibitors, and should be withheld if the patient's blood pressure is low.

5. **Check for accuracy:**

Before submitting your answers, review your choices to ensure that they are accurate and complete. Check if you have selected all the correct options.

Example:
In the heart failure case study scenario, double-check to ensure that all medications that lower blood pressure have been selected, and none that do not affect blood pressure have been chosen.

Let's solve another extended multiple answers question.

QUE: A patient with heart failure is taking multiple medications. Which of the following medications should be withheld if the patient has a low blood pressure reading? Select all that apply.
A) Furosemide
B) Digoxin
C) Lisinopril
D) Spironolactone
E) Metoprolol

Correct Answers:

A) Furosemide C) Lisinopril

Explanation:

   A. Furosemide is a diuretic medication that helps reduce fluid buildup in the body and lower blood pressure. If a patient with heart failure has a low blood pressure reading, withholding furosemide would help avoid a further reduction in blood pressure.

   B) Digoxin is a medication that strengthens the heart's contractions and is used to treat heart failure. However, it does not directly affect blood pressure and does not need to be withheld if a patient has a low blood pressure reading.

   C) Lisinopril is an ACE inhibitor medication that lowers blood pressure and is commonly used to treat heart failure. If a patient has a low blood pressure reading, withholding lisinopril would help avoid a further reduction in blood pressure.

   D) Spironolactone is a potassium-sparing diuretic that helps reduce fluid buildup in the body and lower blood pressure. However, it is not as potent as furosemide in reducing blood pressure, and its use should be evaluated based on the patient's overall condition and clinical presentation.

   E) Metoprolol is a beta-blocker medication that lowers blood pressure and is used to treat heart failure. However, it is not as potent as furosemide or lisinopril in reducing blood pressure, and its use should be evaluated based on the patient's overall condition and clinical presentation.

   In summary, Furosemide and Lisinopril are the correct answers to this question as they are both medications that can significantly reduce blood pressure and should be withheld if the patient has a low blood pressure reading. The other options may also be used to treat heart failure, but do not need to be withheld specifically for low blood pressure.
2. Extended Drag and Drop Questions

"Extended Drag and Drop Questions" refer to a testing method in which instead of merely clicking the correct answer(s), the test-taker must select and drag the correct option(s) to a designated area. This format is particularly useful when testing the ability to prioritize tasks or arrange elements in a specific order.

For instance, a question may ask the test-taker to arrange a list of tasks in order of priority by dragging and dropping each task into the appropriate position. In this way, the test-taker is required to demonstrate their understanding of the relative importance of each task and their ability to organize them accordingly.

By using the drag and drop format, the testing process becomes more interactive and engaging for the test-taker, while also providing a more accurate representation of their knowledge and skills. Overall, the extended drag and drop format offers a unique and effective approach to testing in a variety of contexts.

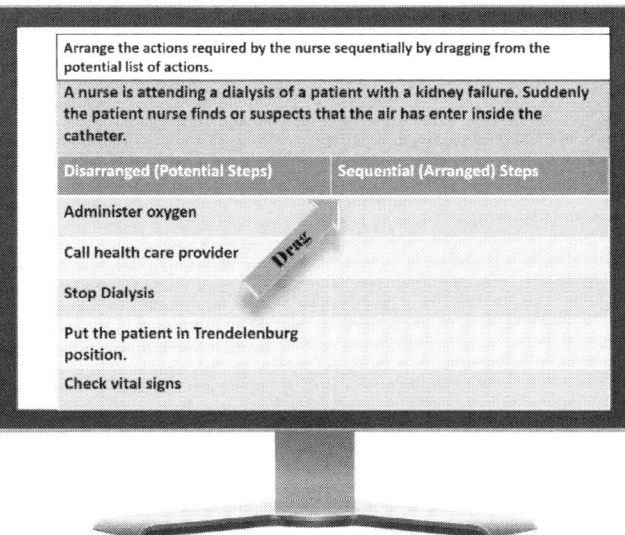

Below are some strategies to effectively approach extended drag-and-drop questions, along with a case study and example of nursing care for a patient who has drowned.

Read the question and instructions carefully: Make sure to read the question stem and any accompanying instructions carefully. These questions can be complex and it is important to understand what is being asked before attempting to answer.

Identify the key concepts: Identify the key concepts or pieces of information that the question is testing. For example, in the case study below, the key concepts might include drowning, nursing care, and patient assessment.

Review all answer options: Read through all answer options carefully, and try to eliminate any that are incorrect. Then, read through the remaining options and consider their relevance to the key concepts identified in step 2.

Determine the correct order: If the question requires the answers to be placed in a specific order, take time to determine the correct order. Often, the order will be provided in the question stem or the instructions.

Practice: Practice is key for mastering extended drag-and-drop questions. Practice answering questions in this format to become comfortable with the process and identify any areas of weakness.

Now, let's look at an example of a case study for nursing care for a patient who has drowned:

Case Study: Nursing Care for Drowning Patient

Mr. Smith, a 54-year-old man, is brought to the emergency department after being pulled from a swimming pool. He is unresponsive and has no pulse. The healthcare team performs cardiopulmonary resuscitation (CPR) and is able to restore a pulse. Mr. Smith is admitted to the hospital and transferred to the medical-surgical unit for ongoing care.

Drag and drop the following nursing interventions in the correct order for Mr. Smith's care:

- Assess Mr. Smith's airway and breathing

- Monitor Mr. Smith's vital signs

- Administer oxygen as needed

- Obtain a chest x-ray to evaluate lung function

- Provide emotional support to Mr. Smith and his family

Answer:

1. Assess Mr. Smith's airway and breathing

2. Administer oxygen as needed

3. Obtain a chest x-ray to evaluate lung function

4. Monitor Mr. Smith's vital signs

5. Provide emotional support to Mr. Smith and his family

Explanation:

In this case, the key concepts are nursing care for a patient who has drowned, and the order of nursing interventions for Mr. Smith's care. The correct order is to first assess Mr. Smith's airway and breathing, then administer oxygen as needed, obtain a chest x-ray to evaluate lung function, monitor vital signs, and finally provide emotional support to Mr. Smith and his family. This order ensures that the most urgent needs are addressed first, followed by ongoing monitoring and emotional support.

3. Cloze Type Questions

Imagine receiving a report that contains several blank spaces, and your task is to fill them with appropriate words or phrases that are missing. These are known as cloze-type questions. One particular type of cloze question involves a report with dropdown options, and you are required to select a phrase that indicates the need for immediate intervention or any actions that need to be taken.

To excel in answering cloze-type questions, you need to have a good understanding of the context and the subject matter. You also need to use your prior knowledge to fill in the gaps accurately. One effective strategy is to eliminate any answer choices that do not fit the context or are unlikely to be correct. For instance, in a cloze-type question that asks you to fill in the blank space in the sentence "I went to the _____ to buy some groceries," you can eliminate the answer "zoo" as it does not fit the context.

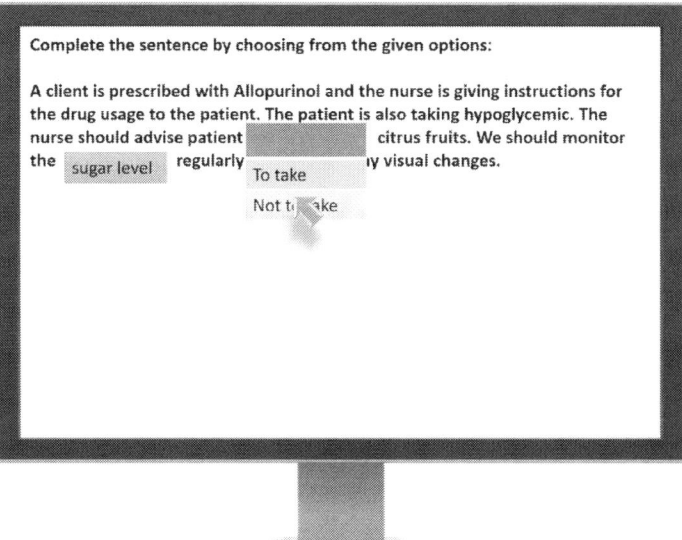

Let's take an example of a nursing care scenario for the lymphatic system to demonstrate how to solve a cloze-type question in the next-generation NCLEX RN exam.

Case Study: Nursing Care for the Lymphatic System

A patient was admitted to the hospital with lymphedema. The nurse caring for the patient should assess the affected limb's size, _____, and skin integrity. The nurse should avoid using tight clothing or _____ on the affected limb, as it can exacerbate the swelling. The nurse should also teach the patient to perform _____ exercises to promote lymphatic drainage.
To solve this cloze-type question, follow these steps:

Read the entire passage or sentence to understand the context and the purpose of the question. In this case, the passage describes nursing care for a patient with lymphedema.

Look for the missing words and phrases, and try to fill them in using your prior knowledge and the context of the passage. For example, in the first sentence, the nurse should assess the affected limb's size, _____, and skin integrity. Based on your prior knowledge of nursing care, you can infer that the missing word is "texture," as it is crucial to assess the texture of the affected limb's skin.

Eliminate answer choices that do not fit. In the second sentence, the nurse should avoid using tight clothing or _____ on the affected limb, as it can exacerbate the swelling. You can eliminate the answer choices that do not make sense in the context of the passage, such as "loose clothing" or "warm compresses." The correct answer is "jewelry," as it can be tight-fitting and put pressure on the affected limb.

Use your prior knowledge and the context of the passage to fill in the remaining missing words or phrases. For example, in the third sentence, the nurse should also teach the patient to perform _____ exercises to promote lymphatic drainage. You can infer that the missing word is "range-of-motion," as exercises that involve moving the affected limb can help promote lymphatic drainage.

So, to solve cloze-type questions in the next-generation NCLEX RN exam, it's essential to read the passage or sentence carefully, use your prior knowledge and the context of the question, and eliminate answer choices that do not fit. By following these steps, you can approach cloze-type questions effectively and increase your chances of getting the correct answer.

4. Matrix / Grid Type Question

A matrix or grid type question is a structured question that is often used in various assessments and exams, including nursing exams like NCLEX RN. These questions are presented in the form of a table or grid with rows and columns, where each row and column represents a unique aspect that needs to be evaluated or matched.

For instance, in a nursing exam, a matrix question could be presented in the form of a table, where the rows contain information about a patient's medical conditions or actions of nurses, while the columns represent options for correct and incorrect answers.

To effectively answer a matrix question, it is crucial to carefully read the instructions and fully comprehend what is being asked. One should also pay close attention to the headings of each row and column, as they provide vital information that helps in evaluating the question.

For example, let's consider a matrix question that is presented in the form of a table with four columns. The first column represents a patient's medical condition, such as hypertension or diabetes, while the other three columns represent different treatment options. In this case, the respondent would need to evaluate each row and match the patient's medical condition with the appropriate treatment option.

Therefore, to answer a matrix question accurately, it is essential to have a clear understanding of the subject matter and carefully evaluate each aspect presented in the table or grid.

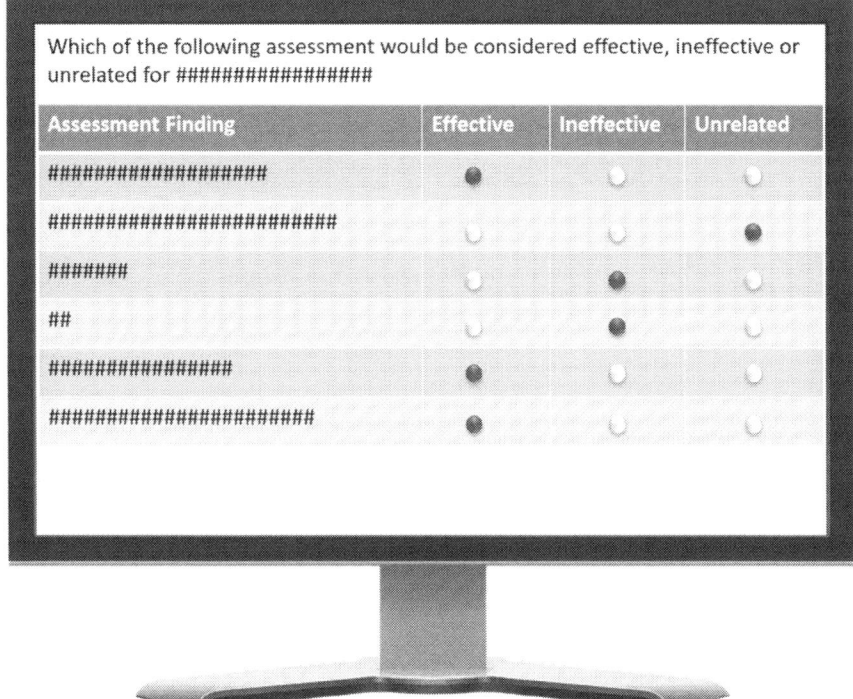

Case study: Ms. Jones is a 65-year-old patient who was admitted to the hospital with complaints of abdominal pain, nausea, and vomiting. She has a history of peptic ulcer disease and takes proton pump inhibitors to manage her symptoms. The physician has ordered a clear liquid diet for Ms. Jones until her symptoms improve.

Instructions: Evaluate the nursing interventions listed below and place them in the appropriate category based on their effectiveness for managing Ms. Jones' digestive symptoms.

In this example, the nursing interventions are listed in the first column, and the headings for each category (effective, ineffective, and unrelated) are listed in the top row. To answer the question, you would need to evaluate each nursing intervention and determine whether it is effective, ineffective, or unrelated for managing Ms. Jones' digestive symptoms.
Here are some possible answers for each nursing intervention:

- Administering antiemetic medication: Effective

- Encouraging Ms. Jones to ambulate in the hallway: Unrelated

- Providing clear liquid diet as ordered: Effective

- Administering antacid medication: Effective

- Instructing Ms. Jones to avoid caffeine and alcohol: Effective

- Applying a heating pad to Ms. Jones' abdomen: Ineffective

As you can see, the effective interventions are those that are likely to improve Ms. Jones' digestive symptoms, while the ineffective interventions are those that are unlikely to improve her symptoms or may even make them worse. The unrelated interventions are those that do not have a direct impact on Ms. Jones' digestive symptoms.

To prepare for matrix questions on the NCLEX RN exam, it's important to review nursing interventions for different patient scenarios and practice categorizing them based on their effectiveness. You can also review sample NCLEX RN exam questions to get a better idea of how matrix questions are structured and what types of nursing interventions may be included in them.

Highlighting

The process of selecting an answer in this context involves highlighting the relevant text or sentences within a medical report. For instance, if you are presented with a medical or patient history report, you will need to carefully examine the document and identify the words and phrases that relate to the question being asked. This approach allows you to pinpoint specific details that are essential to answering the question accurately.

To illustrate this process, imagine you are tasked with identifying the cause of a patient's chronic back pain. You are given access to their medical history, which includes details about their past injuries and surgeries, as well as their current medications and symptoms. To answer the question, you would need to carefully read through the medical report and highlight the relevant information, such as previous back surgeries, ongoing pain management medications, and any recent changes in their symptoms. By selecting these key phrases, you can identify the potential underlying causes of the patient's back pain and provide an accurate diagnosis.

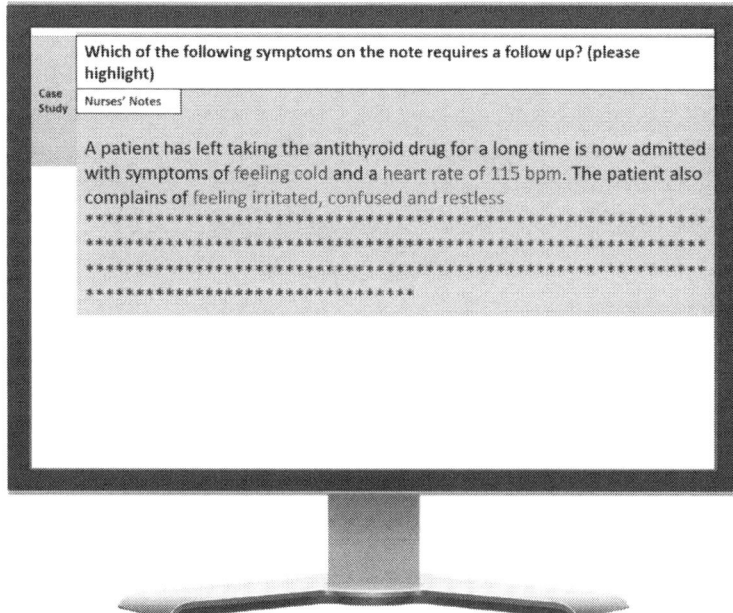

Multiple Choice Questions

The NCLEX examination features a multitude of questions, with a significant proportion falling under the multiple-choice category. As a test taker, you can employ several strategies to ensure that you answer these questions effectively. One such strategy that we will delve into in our lecture on priority-based questions is the use of tricks that can aid you in selecting the correct answer.

To begin with, it is advisable to avoid selecting the option that suggests calling the healthcare provider if the issue can be resolved by a nurse. This is especially important when the situation calls for quick action to save the life of the patient. By opting for this answer choice, you risk wasting time that could be used to provide prompt care to the patient.

Additionally, you should be cautious when faced with answer choices that read "all of the above" or "none of the above." These options are often a trap for test-takers who may be inclined to choose them as a shortcut to save time. It is crucial to read the question carefully and look out for keywords such as "next" or "first" to determine the correct answer.

Another tip is to focus on specific nursing procedures. For instance, when presented with an arterial blood gas (ABG) related question, you should first prioritize the airways, then breathing, and lastly, circulation.

This will help you to determine the appropriate sequence of actions to follow and arrive at the correct answer.

Lastly, it is essential to bear in mind Maslow's hierarchy of needs when answering questions related to the patient's specific needs. The hierarchy prioritizes physiological needs over safety needs, esteem needs, and the need for the patient to feel good. By adhering to this hierarchy, you can arrive at the correct answer.

To gain a more in-depth understanding of these tips, we will provide you with detailed examples during our lecture on prioritizing answers. While these tips are just the basics, they can help you make more informed decisions when selecting answers for multiple-choice questions.
Example:

A patient has been diagnosed with respiratory acidosis based on an ABG test. Which of the following is likely to have caused the acidosis?

A) Damage to the alveoli
B) Hyperventilation
C) Normal carbon dioxide levels in the blood
D) High oxygen saturation in the blood

Answer: A) Damage to the alveoli

Rationale:
Respiratory acidosis is caused by excess carbon dioxide in the body, which can occur when there is damage to the alveoli, resulting in a decreased ability for carbon dioxide to escape from the body.

Explanation: When there is damage to the alveoli it can lead to an excess of carbon dioxide in the body that can react with water to form carbonic acid, causing an acidic environment. Option A) Damage to the alveoli is therefore the most likely cause of the acidosis in this case. Option B) Hyperventilation would actually cause respiratory alkalosis, and options C) Normal carbon dioxide levels in the blood and D) High oxygen saturation in the blood are not relevant causes of respiratory acidosis.

Figure Questions

In these types of questions, you are given a figure which could be a graph or picture.
Generally, I would suggest you give proper emphasis to the EKG interpretation chapter as a lot of probable questions of this type may come based on what you learn there.
Sometimes, you may also be asked to point out or select the definite part of the figure to choose the correct answer.

Example:

A patient is showing a symptom of an extremely high heart rate of around 250 BPM, low BP, shortness of breath, etc. Upon monitoring via cardiac telemetry, the EKG reading shows the 'saw tooth' appearance with multiple P waves for each QRS complex. Can you identify the cardiac condition of this patient?

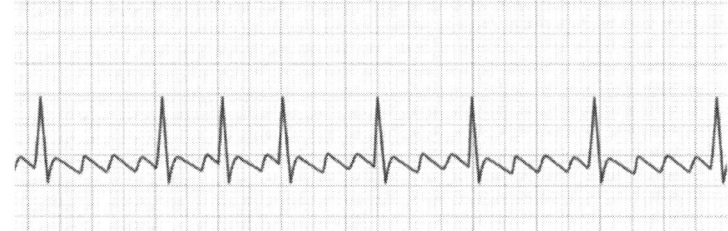

- i.   The EKG shows Atrial Flutter
- ii. The EKG shows Atrial Fibrillation
- iii. This is a Normal sinus
- iv. EKG shows Sinus Bradycardia

Let's first start with the elimination strategy.
Let's see the options. We are given here that the heart rate is very high at around 250 BPM, so the term bradycardia which means low heartbeat of fewer than 60 beats per minute should be eliminated.
We are left with 3 options, 1, 2, and 3. Again, as an elimination strategy, it's too easy to point out that this is not a normal sinus rhythm. The normal sinus rhythm contains normal P wave, QRS complex, and T wave. Normal sinus is the rhythm of a normal person. Is the patient's condition normal here?
No, the symptoms and the nature of ekg strip are not normal so we have to eliminate this one.
We are now left with options 1 and 2.
This question needs specialized knowledge.
If you are new to interpreting the EKG waves. Don't worry. We will practice that with lots of case studies and examples in the relevant section. Just for your knowledge,
In atrial flutter, there is a coordinated electrical activity in the heart. The rate is regular which means the waves look regular but the p wave shows a saw tooth pattern like the one shown in this graph.
So, the correct answer to this question is option 1 or atrial flutter.
Next for option 2, in atrial fibrillation, there is no coordinated electrical activity. The P waves are absent and blunt waves are seen.
The ecg wave or ekg wave looks something like this. Note in this figure that unlike in atrial flutter, there is no regular rhythm and p waves are absent. There are wavy structures that we cannot distinguish from any kind of wave.

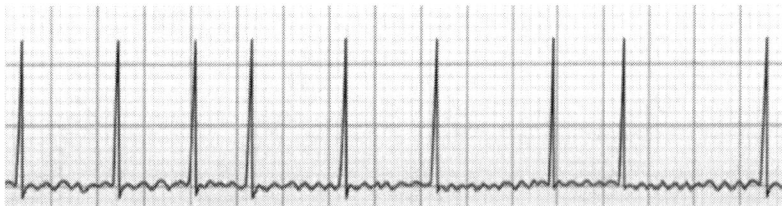

Chart/Table Type Questions

Here, you will be given a chart with some description that may contain the right or the wrong options. You will be prompted to choose the right or wrong options based on the situation.

Example:

A nurse notes down the following symptoms of the patient.
1. the patient has severe hypotension
2. there is a progressive stupor or coma
3. Has electrolyte imbalance upon investigation (decreased sodium level, increased potassium, decreased cortisol, etc)
4. There is dehydration and hypovolemia

Which of these pairs (column) could be correct for the diagnosis and management of this condition?

Diagnosis	Primary Management
Addisonian crisis	IV hydrocortisone
Addison's disease	Hormone Replacement
Cushing syndrome	Potassium Sparing diuretics (Spironolactone)
Cushing syndrome	Hormone Replacement

So, in this question, you have these 4 pairs for the type of disease diagnosis and primary management. The correct answer for this is option no, 1. This is the Addisonian crisis.

Just for your quick knowledge,

Addison's disease is a condition in which there is hypo secretion of adrenocortical hormone and in which the patient shows the following condition. You can memorize this as a 3s condition.

The blood profile shows salt or electrolyte imbalance, there is Sugar or metabolic imbalance and there is sexual imbalance.

Cushing syndrome is hypersecretion of adrenocortical hormone and basically, the symptoms of diabetes are common in cushing syndrome. As a memory tip, understand that there is a 3P-

  i. **Polydipsia** or increase in hunger,
 ii. **Polyuria** or increase in urination,
iii. **Polyphagia** or increase in appetite etc.

Addisonian crisis is a life-threatening emergency of Addison's disease which comes with all the conditions mentioned in the question like
- ✓ severe hypotension
- ✓ progressive stupor or coma
- ✓ electrolyte imbalance upon investigation (decreased sodium level, increased potassium, decreased cortisol, etc.)
- ✓ dehydration and hypovolemia, etc.

26

The primary management of this condition is IV hydrocortisone. If you are asked how to administer hydrocortisone, two third the dose should be given in AM and one-third of the dose is given in PM to mimic the normal diurnal rhythm of the body.
We then taper the dose and withdraw.
So, your option for this question is quite clear. You have to select the first option.

Fill in the blanks type question

Although multiple-choice and other types of questions are more common in the NCLEX examination, you may still encounter fill-in-the-blank questions. These types of questions typically require you to input a specific answer or phrase to complete a sentence or solve a problem.

One common type of fill-in-the-blank question is the calculation-based question, which involves solving mathematical problems related to dosage calculations or other areas of nursing practice. For instance, you may be given a scenario where a patient requires a certain medication dosage, and you need to calculate the correct amount to administer. To answer the question, you would need to input the numerical answer in the blank space provided.

In some cases, you may also be required to round up your answer to a certain number of decimal places. To do this, you can follow some simple rules. For instance, if you need to round up to one decimal place, you should round the number to the nearest tenth. If the digit after the tenths place is five or greater, you should round up to the next highest whole number. For example, if the calculation is 3.87 and you need to round up to one decimal place, the correct answer would be 3.9, not 3.8.

If you need to round up to two decimal places, you should round the number to the nearest hundredth. Again, if the digit after the hundredths place is five or greater, you should round up to the next highest whole number. For instance, if the calculation is 2.463 and you need to round up to two decimal places, the correct answer would be 2.46.

Strategy to ace the fill in the blanks type question

To successfully answer fill in the blanks type questions in the Next Generation NCLEX RN Exam, there are several strategies that can be employed.

Firstly, it is important to read the entire question carefully. This involves paying close attention to the wording of the question and understanding the context in which the missing word is to be inserted. By doing so, you can identify any clues or hints that may help you select the correct answer. For example, if the question is related to a medical condition, you can look for any keywords or phrases that may provide a hint as to what type of word would fit in the blank.

Once you have read the question, the next step is to identify the missing word. This involves determining what type of word would fit in the blank based on the context of the sentence. For instance, if the blank appears in the middle of a sentence and the surrounding words are verbs, it is likely that the missing word is also a verb.

After identifying the missing word, the next step is to review the provided options. This involves carefully analyzing each option and eliminating any that do not fit the context of the sentence. By doing so, you can narrow down your options and increase your chances of selecting the correct answer.

To further increase your chances of selecting the correct answer, it is important to apply your knowledge of the subject matter and use your critical thinking skills. For example, if the question is related to a medical condition, you can use your knowledge of the condition to determine which word would make the most sense in the given sentence. Additionally, you can use your critical thinking skills to determine which word would fit grammatically and logically in the sentence.

Lastly, before submitting your answer, it is important to double-check to ensure that the word you selected fits grammatically and logically in the sentence. This involves reviewing the sentence as a whole and ensuring that the selected word makes sense in the context of the sentence.

Example (Non-Numerical)
Dr. Smith is a pediatrician who is conducting a neonatal assessment of a newborn baby. As part of the assessment, Dr. Smith checks for various physical and reflex characteristics. During the examination, Dr. Smith notices that the baby is lacking _____ on the entire sole of the feet. What could be the potential implications of this observation?

Fill in the blank type question: What physical characteristic is typically absent in premature or genetically disordered newborns?
A) Babinski reflex
B) Epstein's pearl
C) Lanugo hair
D) Planter creases
Answer: D) Planter creases.

Explanation: Planter creases are present on the entire sole of a newborn, and their absence may indicate prematurity or a genetic disorder. Therefore, the correct answer is option D. Babinski reflex, Epstein's pearl, and lanugo hair are all physical characteristics that may be present in newborns, but their presence or absence does not necessarily indicate prematurity or a genetic disorder.

A) Babinski reflex: The Babinski reflex is a primitive reflex that is present in newborns. It is elicited by stroking the lateral surface of the sole of the foot, which causes the toes to hyperextend and fan out. This reflex is normally present in newborns and typically disappears around 12 months of age. The presence or absence of the Babinski reflex can be an indicator of neurologic health in a newborn. In some cases, the Babinski reflex may persist beyond infancy, which can be a sign of a neurologic disorder.

B) Epstein's pearl: Epstein's pearl is a white, pearl-like epithelial cyst that can appear on the gums or palate of newborns. These cysts are harmless and typically disappear within a few weeks after birth. Epstein's pearls are caused by trapped epithelial cells during the development of the baby's mouth.

C) Lanugo hair: Lanugo hair is fine, downy hair that covers the entire body of some newborns. This hair is typically present on premature infants and usually disappears by the time the baby reaches full term. Lanugo hair is thought to help regulate the baby's body temperature and protect their skin in utero.

D) Planter creases: Planter creases are the lines or creases that appear on the entire sole of the feet of newborns. These creases are formed during fetal development and are present in most newborns. The absence of planter creases on the entire sole of the feet may indicate prematurity or a genetic disorder, such as Down syndrome. However, the absence of planter creases alone is not enough to diagnose a disorder and further evaluation and testing would be needed to confirm any potential issues.

Case Study: A 65-year-old patient with a history of hypertension and type 2 diabetes mellitus is admitted to the hospital with complaints of shortness of breath and chest pain. Upon examination, the healthcare provider notes an elevated blood pressure of 170/95 mmHg and a blood glucose level of 250 mg/dL.

Question: The healthcare provider should administer _____ to the patient to lower the blood pressure.

A. Insulin
B. Amlodipine
C. Metformin
D. Lisinopril

Strategy:

Read the entire question carefully: In this case, the question asks which medication the healthcare provider should administer to lower the patient's blood pressure.

Identify the missing word: The blank is asking for the name of the medication.

Review the provided options: There are four options given: Insulin, Amlodipine, Metformin, and Lisinopril. Based on the context of the sentence, Insulin and Metformin are unlikely to be the correct options since they are used to treat diabetes, not hypertension.

Use your knowledge and critical thinking skills: Amlodipine and Lisinopril are both medications used to treat hypertension. However, in this case, Lisinopril may be the better option since it is an ACE inhibitor and can also help protect the kidneys, which is important in patients with diabetes.

Double-check your answer: Before submitting your answer, double-check to make sure the word "Lisinopril" fits grammatically and logically in the sentence. The sentence should read: "The healthcare provider should administer Lisinopril to the patient to lower the blood pressure."

Some Important Case Study Question Solving Strategies

1. Introduction of Case Studies
The N G N introduces case studies to better assess a candidate's ability to make clinical judgments and think critically. Unlike traditional exams that focus on recalling information, these case studies simulate real-world situations that nurses face in their practice. For example, you may be given a scenario involving a postoperative patient with abnormal vital signs, requiring you to analyze the situation, make decisions, and prioritize actions.

2. Three Case Studies
Each NGN exam includes three scored case studies, each containing six related questions, making up a total of 18 questions. These case studies cover different clinical scenarios, ensuring a comprehensive evaluation of a nurse's ability to manage a variety of patient conditions. For instance, one case may involve a pediatric patient with respiratory distress, while another focuses on an elderly patient with heart failure.

3. Unfolding Scenarios
Case studies use an "unfolding" format, where patient information is gradually revealed in stages. This mirrors how information is often received in clinical practice and requires candidates to adapt as new data becomes available. For example, you might initially receive basic patient details, but as the case progresses, you may learn about unexpected lab results or worsening symptoms that change the clinical picture. On this book, you are provided with many case study questions with unfolding scenario. These are not meant to confuse you but mimic the real practice environment.

4. Clinical Judgment Measurement Model
Questions in the case studies are based on the NCSBN Clinical Judgment Measurement Model (CJMM). This framework assesses how nurses collect and analyze data, make decisions, and implement interventions. For instance, a question might ask you to prioritize interventions for a patient with sepsis, following the CJMM steps of recognizing and analyzing clinical cues.
The CJMM outlines six key steps that nurses follow when providing patient care:
- Recognize Cues: Identify relevant patient information (e.g., vital signs, symptoms, lab results).
- Analyze Cues: Interpret the data to understand its significance and implications for the patient's condition.
- Prioritize Hypotheses: Determine the most likely explanations or diagnoses based on the cues.
- Generate Solutions: Develop appropriate interventions or actions to address the patient's needs.
- Take Action: Implement the chosen interventions effectively.
- Evaluate Outcomes: Assess whether the interventions were successful and adjust care as needed.

5. Multiple Question Types
NGN case studies incorporate various question types, such as multiple response, drag-and-drop, drop-down, highlight, and matrix/grid questions. These formats test different aspects of clinical reasoning and decision-making. For example, you might be asked to drag and drop the correct sequence of interventions for a patient experiencing a stroke.

6. Realistic Scenarios
The scenarios presented in case studies are designed to mimic real-life nursing situations, ensuring that the exam evaluates practical skills. For instance, a scenario about a patient with congestive heart failure might involve managing fluid balance, adjusting medications, and interpreting lab results over several days.

7. Layered Information

Case studies provide information in layers, including nurse's notes, medical history, and vital signs, requiring candidates to synthesize data from multiple sources. For example, a patient's increased blood pressure may first be noted in progress notes, followed by lab data showing decreased kidney function, all of which must be considered together to determine the next steps.

8. Critical Thinking
The NGN case studies demand higher-level critical thinking skills compared to traditional multiple-choice questions. Candidates must analyze complex situations, interpret data, and make well-reasoned decisions. For example, managing a postoperative patient with unexpected bleeding requires more than recalling textbook knowledge; it demands real-time assessment and action.

9. Partial Credit Scoring
Unlike traditional exams, NGN case studies use partial credit scoring, allowing candidates to earn points for partially correct answers. This system recognizes nuanced understanding. For example, if you correctly identify two out of three necessary interventions for a patient in shock, you may still earn partial credit.

10. Pathophysiology Focus
A deeper understanding of pathophysiology is essential for analyzing case studies effectively. This knowledge helps candidates link clinical signs to underlying disease processes. For instance, understanding how diabetic ketoacidosis affects electrolytes and blood pH can guide decisions about treatment priorities.

CASE STUDY 1 : Clinical Presentation of Parkinson's Disease

History:

65-year-old female
Gradual onset of tremors and stiffness over the past two years
Family history of neurodegenerative disorders

Assessment:

Motor Symptoms:

Resting tremors
Bradykinesia
Rigidity
Postural instability

Non-Motor Symptoms:
Sleep disturbances
Occasional depressive episodes
Intact cognitive function with occasional memory lapses

Vital Signs:

Blood Pressure: 130/80 mmHg
Heart Rate: 72 bpm
Respiratory Rate: 18 breaths per minute

Medications:

Levodopa: 100 mg TID
Pramipexole: 0.5 mg QD
Rasagiline: 1 mg QD
Trihexyphenidyl: 2 mg PRN for tremors

Que 1: What is the most likely condition the patient is suffering from based on the provided information?

A) Alzheimer's disease
B) Essential Tremor
C) Parkinson's disease
D) Multiple sclerosis
E) Huntington's disease

Ans 1-Explanation:

Correct Answer: C) Parkinson's disease

Reasoning:

Gradual Onset of Tremors and Stiffness: The patient has a gradual onset of tremors and stiffness over the past two years. This is characteristic of Parkinson's disease, which is a progressive neurodegenerative disorder affecting movement.

Family History of Neurodegenerative Disorders: The patient has a family history of neurodegenerative disorders, which may increase the likelihood of Parkinson's disease.

Motor Symptoms:

Resting Tremors: The presence of resting tremors is a key feature of Parkinson's disease.
Bradykinesia: Slow movement is a characteristic motor symptom of Parkinson's disease.
Rigidity: Muscle stiffness is another common motor symptom in Parkinson's disease.
Postural Instability: The patient exhibits postural instability, which is often seen in advanced stages of Parkinson's disease.
Non-Motor Symptoms:

Sleep Disturbances: Common in Parkinson's disease.
Occasional Depressive Episodes: Depression is a non-motor symptom associated with Parkinson's disease.
Intact Cognitive Function with Occasional Memory Lapses: Cognitive function is generally preserved in Parkinson's disease, but occasional memory lapses may occur.

Vital Signs:

Blood Pressure, Heart Rate, Respiratory Rate: Within normal range, which is typical in Parkinson's disease.
Incorrect Options:

A) Alzheimer's Disease: Alzheimer's disease primarily affects cognition, and the patient in the case study does not exhibit significant cognitive decline.

B) Essential Tremor: Essential tremor typically involves isolated tremors without the presence of other Parkinsonian motor symptoms like bradykinesia and rigidity.

D) Multiple Sclerosis: Multiple sclerosis is a demyelinating disorder that primarily affects the central nervous system but does not present with the typical parkinsonian motor symptoms seen in the case.

E) Huntington's Disease: Huntington's disease is characterized by chorea (involuntary movements), psychiatric symptoms, and cognitive decline, which are not evident in the patient's presentation.

Que 2: Considering the case study of a 65-year-old female with Parkinson's disease symptoms, which vital sign might require monitoring closely due to the prescribed medications?

A) Heart Rate: 72 bpm

B) Respiratory Rate: 18 breaths per minute

C) Blood Pressure: 140/90 mmHg

D) Heart Rate: 80 bpm

D) Respiratory Rate: 16 breaths per minute

E) Blood Pressure: 120/75 mmHg

F) Heart Rate: 65 bpm

Ans 2:

Correct Answer: C) Blood Pressure: 140/90 mmHg

Explanation:

Blood Pressure: 140/90 mmHg (Option C): Hypertension is a potential side effect of both levodopa and pramipexole. Regular monitoring of blood pressure is crucial to identify and manage any hypertensive effects.

Incorrect Options:

Heart Rate: 72 bpm (Option A): While levodopa can cause cardiovascular side effects, changes in heart rate are not as commonly associated with its use.

Respiratory Rate: 18 breaths per minute (Option B): Parkinson's disease medications are not typically associated with significant changes in respiratory rate.

Heart Rate: 80 bpm (Option D): Similar to Option A, changes in heart rate are not a primary concern with the medications mentioned in the case study.

Respiratory Rate: 16 breaths per minute (Option E): Respiratory rate is not directly influenced by the medications used for Parkinson's disease.

Blood Pressure: 120/75 mmHg (Option F): While monitoring blood pressure is important, the options with blood pressure values outside the normal range are more relevant due to the potential hypertensive effects of the medications.

Heart Rate: 65 bpm (Option G): Changes in heart rate are not a primary concern with the medications mentioned in the case study.

Que 3: Which of the following statements by the nurse is NOT accurate regarding the nursing management of Parkinson's disease in the presented case?

A. "The patient's family history of neurodegenerative disorders may have contributed to the development of Parkinson's disease."
B. "The nurse should monitor the patient for postural instability as it is a common motor symptom of Parkinson's disease."
C. "Levodopa is prescribed three times a day to help manage the motor symptoms of Parkinson's disease."
D. "Pramipexole, a dopamine agonist, is administered once daily to improve motor function."
E. "Rasagiline, an MAO-B inhibitor, is prescribed once daily to slow down the progression of Parkinson's disease."
F. "Trihexyphenidyl is given as needed (PRN) for tremors to provide quick relief during exacerbations."
G. "The patient's intact cognitive function with occasional memory lapses indicates effective management of non-motor symptoms."
H. "Sleep disturbances and depressive episodes are common non-motor symptoms that the nurse should assess and address."

Ans 3- G. "The patient's intact cognitive function with occasional memory lapses indicates effective management of non-motor symptoms."

Explanation:

A. "The patient's family history of neurodegenerative disorders may have contributed to the development of Parkinson's disease."

This is accurate. A family history of neurodegenerative disorders can increase the likelihood of developing Parkinson's disease.

B. "The nurse should monitor the patient for postural instability as it is a common motor symptom of Parkinson's disease."

This is accurate. Postural instability is indeed a common motor symptom of Parkinson's disease, especially in the advanced stages.

C. "Levodopa is prescribed three times a day to help manage the motor symptoms of Parkinson's disease."

This is accurate. Levodopa is a standard medication for managing motor symptoms in Parkinson's disease and is typically taken multiple times a day.

D. "Pramipexole, a dopamine agonist, is administered once daily to improve motor function."

This is accurate. Pramipexole is a dopamine agonist used to improve motor function in Parkinson's disease and can be administered once daily.

E. "Rasagiline, an MAO-B inhibitor, is prescribed once daily to slow down the progression of Parkinson's disease."

This is accurate. Rasagiline is an MAO-B inhibitor used to slow down the progression of Parkinson's disease and is taken once daily.

F. "Trihexyphenidyl is given as needed (PRN) for tremors to provide quick relief during exacerbations."

This is accurate. Trihexyphenidyl can be given as needed (PRN) for tremors to provide quick relief during exacerbations.

G. "The patient's intact cognitive function with occasional memory lapses indicates effective management of non-motor symptoms."

This statement is not accurate. Occasional memory lapses may still indicate that non-motor symptoms are present and may require further assessment and management.

H. "Sleep disturbances and depressive episodes are common non-motor symptoms that the nurse should assess and address."

This is accurate. Sleep disturbances and depressive episodes are common non-motor symptoms of Parkinson's disease, and the nurse should assess and address them.

Therefore, the statement that is NOT accurate regarding the nursing management of Parkinson's disease in the presented case is G. "The patient's intact cognitive function with occasional memory lapses indicates effective management of non-motor symptoms."

Que 4: Fill in the blanks with correct answer choice:

Parkinson's disease primarily results from the degeneration of _____ in the brain. There are two primary types of Parkinson's disease: idiopathic or primary Parkinson's, which has no identifiable cause, and secondary Parkinsonism, which occurs as a result of other medical conditions, such as certain medications or head injuries. Non-motor symptoms of Parkinson's disease include sleep disturbances, depression, cognitive impairment, and autonomic dysfunction.

Options:

Neurotransmitters
Neurons
Synapses
Receptors
Axons

Ans 4-Explanation:

The correct answers are 2. Neurons. Parkinson's disease primarily results from the degeneration of dopamine-producing neurons in the brain. Dopamine is a neurotransmitter that plays a crucial role in movement control, and its deficiency leads to the characteristic motor symptoms of Parkinson's.

Option 1 (Neurotransmitters) is incorrect because it does not specify the degeneration of a particular component responsible for dopamine production.

Options 3 (Synapses), 4 (Receptors), and 5 (Axons) are also incorrect as they are not directly related to the degeneration observed in Parkinson's disease. The key issue lies in the loss of dopamine-producing neurons. Synapses and receptors are involved in neuronal communication, and axons are part of the neuron structure, but the primary issue in Parkinson's disease is the loss of dopamine-producing neurons.

Que 5: Identify the Incorrect Sentence:

Parkinson's disease is a progressive neurological disorder affecting movement control, often caused by the degeneration of dopamine-producing neurons. Symptoms include tremors, bradykinesia, and cognitive impairment. While there's no cure, therapeutic interventions, such as speech therapy and a sedentary lifestyle, can help manage symptoms and improve patients' overall well-being.

Which Sentence is Incorrect?

"Parkinson's disease is a progressive neurological disorder affecting movement control."
"Symptoms include tremors, bradykinesia, and cognitive impairment."
"While there's no cure, therapeutic interventions can help manage symptoms."
"Speech therapy and a sedentary lifestyle can improve patients' overall well-being."
"Parkinson's disease is caused by the degeneration of dopamine-producing neurons."

Ans 5:

Explanation:

The correct answer is 4. "Speech therapy and a sedentary lifestyle can improve patients' overall well-being." This sentence is incorrect because it suggests that a sedentary lifestyle can improve well-being, which is not true. Regular exercise, not a sedentary lifestyle, is essential for managing Parkinson's disease symptoms and enhancing overall health.

Que 6:

Which Row Should be Deleted?

Option	Column 1	Column 2	Column 3
1	Motor Symptoms	Tremors	Associated with Parkinson's Disease
2	Medication Management	Administering medications on time	Part of Parkinson's Disease management
3	Cardiovascular Exercise	Enhancing cardiovascular health	Directly associated with Parkinson's
4	Deep Brain Stimulation	Surgical intervention for advanced cases	Treatment option for advanced Parkinson's
5	Genetic Mutations	Contributing factor to Parkinson's development	Linked to the causes of Parkinson's

3. Cardiovascular Exercise

Explanation:
The correct answer is 3. Cardiovascular Exercise because it is not directly associated with Parkinson's Disease. While exercise, including cardiovascular exercise, is beneficial for overall health, the primary focus in managing Parkinson's disease is on motor symptoms and medication management.

Options 1 and 2 are directly associated with Parkinson's disease, involving symptoms and their management. Option 4, Deep Brain Stimulation, is a surgical intervention for advanced cases of Parkinson's disease. Option 5, Genetic Mutations, is a contributing factor to the development of Parkinson's disease.

CASE STUDY 2: Early Diagnosis and Management of Type 2 Diabetes Mellitus.

Patient Information:

Name: Mr. Pavlo Smith
Age: 55 years
Gender: Male
Occupation: Office Manager
Medical History: Hypertension, Hyperlipidemia

Presenting Complaint:

Mr. Smith presents to the clinic with complaints of increased thirst, frequent urination, and unexplained weight loss over the past few weeks. He reports feeling fatigued and has noticed blurred vision on several occasions.

Nurse's Notes:

History:

Mr. Smith has a medical history significant for hypertension and hyperlipidemia.
No history of major surgeries.
Social history: Non-smoker, occasional alcohol use, sedentary lifestyle.

Physical Examination:

General Appearance: Appears tired, slightly overweight.
Eyes: Fundoscopic exam reveals early signs of diabetic retinopathy.
Skin: Dry skin, no evidence of wounds or infections.
Neurological: No focal deficits, but diminished vibratory sensation in lower extremities.

Vital Signs:

Blood Pressure: 140/90 mmHg
Heart Rate: 82 bpm
Respiratory Rate: 18 breaths/min
Temperature: 98.6°F (37°C)
Oxygen Saturation: 98% on room air

Laboratory Results:

Fasting Blood Glucose: 210 mg/dL (Normal: 70-100 mg/dL)
Hemoglobin A1c: 9.5% (Normal: <5.7%)
Lipid Profile: Elevated LDL cholesterol (160 mg/dL), elevated triglycerides (200 mg/dL), decreased HDL cholesterol (35 mg/dL).
Creatinine: 1.0 mg/dL (Normal: 0.5-1.2 mg/dL)
Urine Analysis: Positive for glucosuria and ketonuria.

Que 1: Based on the provided information, what is the right condition that Mr. Pavlo Smith is likely suffering from?

Hypertension
Hyperlipidemia
Diabetic Retinopathy
Type 2 Diabetes Mellitus
Chronic Kidney Disease

Ans 1:

Correct Answer: 4. Type 2 Diabetes Mellitus

Why it's the right answer:

Mr. Pavlo Smith is likely suffering from Type 2 Diabetes Mellitus based on the following findings:

Increased thirst, frequent urination, and unexplained weight loss are classic symptoms of diabetes.
Fatigue and blurred vision are also common symptoms associated with uncontrolled diabetes.
Elevated fasting blood glucose of 210 mg/dL and a high Hemoglobin A1c of 9.5% indicate poor glycemic control, characteristic of diabetes.
Positive findings in urine analysis for glucosuria and ketonuria further support the diagnosis of diabetes. Note that while both types of diabetes can exhibit glucosuria (glucose in the urine), ketonuria (ketones in the urine) is more commonly linked to Type 1 Diabetes Mellitus or diabetic ketoacidosis (DKA), and is less prevalent in Type 2 diabetes.

The fundoscopic exam revealing early signs of diabetic retinopathy is a complication associated with diabetes.

Hypertension: Mr. Smith has a history of hypertension, but the symptoms (increased thirst, frequent urination, unexplained weight loss) and the abnormal laboratory findings (elevated blood glucose, high Hemoglobin A1c) are more indicative of diabetes.

Hyperlipidemia: While Mr. Smith has hyperlipidemia, the constellation of symptoms and laboratory findings is more suggestive of diabetes.

Diabetic Retinopathy: Diabetic retinopathy is mentioned in the nurse's notes, but it is a complication of diabetes rather than the primary condition causing the symptoms.

Chronic Kidney Disease: While the creatinine level is mentioned and is within the normal range, the symptoms and laboratory findings are more indicative of uncontrolled diabetes rather than chronic kidney disease at this point. However, chronic kidney disease can be a complication of long-term uncontrolled diabetes.

Que 2: Which of the following statements from a nurse is NOT appropriate in the nursing management of a patient with Type 2 Diabetes Mellitus?

Options:

1. "You should aim to maintain a healthy weight through a balanced diet and regular exercise."
2. "It's important to monitor your blood glucose levels regularly to ensure they stay within the target range."
3. "Skipping meals occasionally can help control blood sugar levels."
4. "Take your prescribed medications as directed, even if you feel well."
5. "If you experience symptoms of hypoglycemia, consume a sugary snack or drink to raise your blood sugar."
6. "Smoking cessation is crucial for managing diabetes and reducing cardiovascular risk."
7. "Limit your fluid intake to avoid excessive thirst and urination."

Explanation:

Ans 2:
Answers: 3. "Skipping meals occasionally can help control blood sugar levels." And 7. "Limit your fluid intake to avoid excessive thirst and urination."

Encouraging the patient to skip meals is not appropriate in the management of Type 2 Diabetes Mellitus. Consistent, balanced meals are crucial for managing blood glucose levels. Skipping meals can lead to hypoglycemia or overeating later, causing blood sugar fluctuations.

"Limit your fluid intake to avoid excessive thirst and urination." - Incorrect: While monitoring fluid intake is important, advising strict limitation may not be appropriate. Adequate hydration is generally encouraged unless otherwise contraindicated.

Other options:

"You should aim to maintain a healthy weight through a balanced diet and regular exercise." - Correct: Promoting a healthy weight through diet and exercise is essential for diabetes management.

"It's important to monitor your blood glucose levels regularly to ensure they stay within the target range." - Correct: Regular monitoring helps in maintaining glycemic control and adjusting treatment as needed.

"Take your prescribed medications as directed, even if you feel well." - Correct: Medication adherence is crucial for managing blood glucose levels and preventing complications.

"If you experience symptoms of hypoglycemia, consume a sugary snack or drink to raise your blood sugar." - Correct: This advice is appropriate for managing hypoglycemic episodes.

"Smoking cessation is crucial for managing diabetes and reducing cardiovascular risk." - Correct: Smoking cessation is important for overall cardiovascular health and complements diabetes management.

Que 3: Which of the following statements by the nurse is NOT appropriate in the management of a patient with Type 2 Diabetes Mellitus?

A) "Maintaining a consistent meal schedule is important for stable blood sugar levels."

B) "It's essential to incorporate both aerobic and strength training exercises into your routine."

C) "You should limit your carbohydrate intake to prevent blood sugar spikes."

D) "In case of hyperglycemia, it's important to increase your physical activity immediately."

Answer: The statement that is NOT appropriate is:

D) "In case of hyperglycemia, it's important to increase your physical activity immediately."

Explanation: While physical activity is generally beneficial for managing blood sugar levels, it is not advisable to increase physical activity immediately in the case of hyperglycemia without first assessing the situation and consulting a healthcare provider. Hyperglycemia can sometimes indicate other underlying issues, and an inappropriate response can exacerbate the condition. It's important to follow a structured treatment plan for hyperglycemia, including medication adjustments and dietary changes, as directed by a healthcare professional.

Que 5: Select if the row contains 'correct' or 'incorrect' information:

Management of Diabetes	Explanation
Maintain a healthy weight through diet and exercise.	Regular physical activity and a balanced diet are crucial for managing weight and improving insulin sensitivity in diabetes.
Monitor blood glucose levels regularly.	Regular monitoring helps in understanding and managing blood glucose levels, enabling timely adjustments to treatment plans.
Skipping meals occasionally aids in blood sugar control.	Sometimes when the blood sugar shoots up, skipping meal could be a good choice to keep the level of blood sugar normal.
Take prescribed medications as directed, even if feeling well.	Medication adherence is essential for maintaining stable blood glucose levels and preventing complications associated with diabetes.
Consume a sugary snack to raise blood sugar in case of hypoglycemia.	In the event of low blood sugar, consuming a sugary snack or drink helps raise blood sugar levels and manage hypoglycemic symptoms effectively.
Smoking cessation is crucial for managing diabetes and reducing cardiovascular risk.	Quitting smoking is essential for overall cardiovascular health and complements diabetes management by reducing associated risks.
Limit fluid intake to avoid excessive thirst and urination.	While monitoring fluid intake is important, this statement is incorrect. Adequate hydration is generally encouraged unless otherwise contraindicated in diabetes management.

Which row contains incorrect information in the management of diabetes?

Ans 5:

Explanation:

The row with "Skipping meals occasionally aids in blood sugar control" contains incorrect information. Skipping meals can lead to blood sugar fluctuations, potentially causing hypoglycemia or overeating later. Consistent, balanced meals are crucial for glycemic control in diabetes. All other rows provide accurate guidance for managing diabetes, emphasizing the importance of a healthy lifestyle, regular monitoring, medication adherence, and appropriate responses to hypoglycemic episodes.

Que 6:

Which of the following statements by the patient indicates the need for counseling regarding diabetes management?

Options:

1. "I check my blood glucose levels regularly and record the results in a logbook."
2. "I occasionally forget to take my prescribed diabetes medications."
3. "I engage in moderate-intensity exercise for at least 30 minutes most days of the week."
4. "I follow a well-balanced diet with a mix of carbohydrates, proteins, and healthy fats."
5. "I usually consume sugary snacks between meals to keep my energy up."
6. "I quit smoking as soon as I was diagnosed with diabetes."
7. "I limit my alcohol intake to one drink per day as recommended by my healthcare provider."
8. "I understand the importance of maintaining a healthy weight for managing diabetes."
9. "I skip meals occasionally to control my blood sugar levels."
10. "I have an emergency kit with glucose tablets in case my blood sugar drops unexpectedly."

Ans 6:

Correct Answers:

Option 2: Forgetting to take prescribed diabetes medications can have a significant impact on glycemic control and warrants counseling.
Option 5: Consuming sugary snacks between meals may contribute to blood sugar fluctuations and requires counseling for better dietary choices.
Option 9: Skipping meals to control blood sugar levels is not recommended and necessitates counseling on the importance of regular, balanced meals.

Incorrect Answers:

Options 1, 3, 4, 6, 7, 8, and 10: These statements indicate positive behaviors such as regular monitoring, engaging in exercise, following a balanced diet, quitting smoking, limiting alcohol intake, understanding the importance of maintaining a healthy weight, and being prepared with an emergency kit, respectively. While further education may be beneficial, they do not specifically indicate a need for counseling on diabetes management.

CASE STUDY 3: Challenges and Management of Prolonged Labor in Primigravida

Patient Information:

History:

Sarah, a 27-year-old woman at 39 weeks gestation, presents to the labor and delivery unit with severe abdominal pain and prolonged labor. She reports regular contractions that started approximately 12 hours ago, occurring every 5 minutes. The pain has been intensifying, and she describes it as more severe than during her previous pregnancy.
Medical History: G2P1 (Gravida 2, Para 1), Previous uncomplicated vaginal delivery
Current Pregnancy: Singleton, no known complications

Vital Signs:

Blood Pressure: 130/80 mmHg
Heart Rate: 110 bpm
Respiratory Rate: 18 bpm
Temperature: 37.5°C (99.5°F)
Oxygen Saturation: 98% on room air

Medications:

Epidural Analgesia: Administered 6 hours ago for pain management. Patient reports relief initially but now experiencing increased pain in the lower abdomen.
Oxytocin (Pitocin): Initiated to augment labor progress 8 hours ago, currently infusing at 10 units/hour.

Laboratory Results:

Complete Blood Count (CBC):
Hemoglobin: 11.2 g/dL
Hematocrit: 34%
White Blood Cell Count: 14,000/mm^3
Platelet Count: 220,000/mm^3

QUE 1:

What is the most likely cause of Sarah's increased abdominal pain and prolonged labor despite epidural analgesia and oxytocin infusion?

A) Uterine rupture
B) Maternal dehydration
C) Fetal distress
D) Cervical insufficiency
E) Epidural analgesia failure
F) Oxytocin resistance

Correct Answer: A) Uterine rupture

Ans 1:

In this case, the most likely cause of increased abdominal pain and prolonged labor despite epidural analgesia and oxytocin infusion is uterine rupture. Uterine rupture is a serious complication where there is a tear in the uterine wall, often leading to severe abdominal pain, fetal distress, and prolonged labor. Given Sarah's history of regular contractions, the presence of pain more severe than in her previous pregnancy, and the need for emergency cesarean section due to suspected uterine rupture, option A is the correct answer.

Incorrect Options:

B) Maternal dehydration: While dehydration can contribute to complications in labor, it is not the primary cause of increased abdominal pain and prolonged labor in this case.
C) Fetal distress: Fetal distress could be a consequence of uterine rupture, but it is not the primary cause of the symptoms described.
D) Cervical insufficiency: Cervical insufficiency typically presents with painless cervical dilation and is not the likely cause of severe abdominal pain in this scenario.
E) Epidural analgesia failure: While epidural analgesia may fail to provide complete pain relief, it is unlikely to be the sole cause of increased abdominal pain and prolonged labor.
F) Oxytocin resistance: Oxytocin resistance could contribute to labor complications, but it is not the primary cause of the symptoms described.

Que 2:

Emergency Cesarean Section: The obstetrician performs a thorough assessment and decides to proceed with an emergency cesarean section due to suspected uterine rupture.

Postoperative Care: Sarah undergoes repair of the uterine rupture during the cesarean section. Postoperatively, she receives additional blood transfusions and antibiotics.

Monitoring: Both the mother and the baby are closely monitored in the postpartum period.

Follow-Up Care: Appropriate support and follow-up care are provided to ensure the well-being of both the mother and the newborn.

MCQ Question:

Which intervention is not directly mentioned in the case as part of the management for suspected uterine rupture?

A) Emergency Cesarean Section
B) Blood Transfusions
C) Antibiotics
D) Induction of Labor

Ans 2:
Correct Answer: D) Induction of Labor

Explanation:

A) Emergency Cesarean Section: The obstetrician decides to proceed with an emergency cesarean section due to suspected uterine rupture. This is directly mentioned in the case and is a crucial intervention for addressing the identified complication.

B) Blood Transfusions: Postoperatively, Sarah receives additional blood transfusions. This is mentioned as part of the management to address the potential maternal hemorrhage associated with uterine rupture.

C) Antibiotics: Sarah receives antibiotics postoperatively, which is a standard practice to prevent or treat infection, especially in the context of uterine rupture.

D) Induction of Labor: Induction of labor is not mentioned in the case as part of the interventions for suspected uterine rupture. In fact, the case describes that Sarah was already in labor, and the focus was on addressing the complications associated with the ongoing labor.

QUE 3:

After the birth, the nurse provides crucial advice to the patient for optimal postpartum recovery. First and foremost, the nurse emphasizes the importance of proper hygiene to prevent infections, advising the patient to keep the perineal area clean and dry. Additionally, the nurse recommends a well-balanced diet rich in nutrients to support the healing process and breastfeeding, if applicable. Adequate rest and sleep are stressed, encouraging the new mother to nap when the baby sleeps. The nurse also educates on postpartum exercises to aid in regaining strength and tone. Proper hydration is highlighted, advocating for increased water intake. Furthermore, the nurse advises against heavy lifting during the initial weeks and suggests the use of a supportive abdominal binder for added comfort. Lastly, the importance of emotional well-being is underscored, promoting open communication and seeking support when needed.

Highlight the Incorrect Sentences:

Ans 3:

"Adequate rest and sleep are stressed, encouraging the new mother to nap when the baby sleeps."

Correct: Adequate rest and sleep are crucial for postpartum recovery, and napping when the baby sleeps is a practical suggestion to ensure the mother gets sufficient rest.

"The nurse also educates on postpartum exercises to aid in regaining strength and tone."

Incorrect: Postpartum exercises are generally recommended, but this sentence is vague. It doesn't specify the type or intensity of exercises, which should be individualized and approved by a healthcare professional.

"Proper hydration is highlighted, advocating for increased water intake."

Correct: Proper hydration is crucial for postpartum recovery, especially for breastfeeding mothers. Increased water intake supports overall health and aids in milk production.

"The nurse advises against heavy lifting during the initial weeks."

Correct: Avoiding heavy lifting is important during the initial weeks postpartum to prevent strain on the body as it heals.

"The nurse recommends a well-balanced diet rich in nutrients to support the healing process and breastfeeding, if applicable."

Correct: A well-balanced diet is essential for postpartum recovery and breastfeeding mothers, providing the necessary nutrients for healing and milk production.

"The nurse emphasizes the importance of proper hygiene to prevent infections, advising the patient to keep the perineal area clean and dry."

Correct: Proper hygiene is crucial to prevent infections, and keeping the perineal area clean and dry is an effective preventive measure.

"The nurse advises the use of a supportive abdominal binder for added comfort."

Incorrect: The use of an abdominal binder is a controversial topic. Some healthcare professionals discourage its routine use, as it may interfere with natural abdominal muscle recovery. Individual assessment and guidance are necessary.

"Additionally, the nurse recommends a well-balanced diet rich in nutrients to support the healing process and breastfeeding, if applicable."

Correct: Reiterating the importance of a well-balanced diet emphasizes its significance in the postpartum period, catering to both healing and potential breastfeeding.

"The importance of emotional well-being is underscored, promoting open communication and seeking support when needed."

Correct: Addressing emotional well-being is crucial postpartum, and promoting open communication and seeking support contribute to a healthier mental state for the new mother.

QUE 4:

Contraindications	Nursing Management	Incorrect?
Maternal Hypertension	Monitor blood pressure regularly.	
Allergy to Oxytocin	Administer Pitocin cautiously, under the supervision of healthcare provider.	
Placenta Previa	Avoid vaginal examinations. Continuous fetal monitoring.	
Active Herpes Infection	C-section recommended to prevent neonatal exposure.	
Gestational Diabetes	Monitor blood glucose levels regularly. Encourage a balanced diet.	
Previous Uterine Surgery	Assess for signs of uterine rupture during labor. Consider the risk of scar dehiscence.	
Eclampsia	Administer magnesium sulfate as prescribed. Monitor for signs of seizures.	

Identify the Incorrect Row:

Ans 4:

Incorrect Row: "Allergy to Oxytocin"
Explanation: While the nursing management advises administering Pitocin cautiously under the supervision of a healthcare provider, this might not be applicable for a patient with a known allergy to Oxytocin. Allergic reactions can be severe, and in such cases, alternative strategies or medications should be considered, making this row incorrect.

QUE 5:

Which of the following statements by the nurse is NOT indicative of potential complications in Sarah Johnson's labor and delivery?

"The fetal heart rate is monitored continuously, and it is within the normal range."
"Sarah's white blood cell count is elevated, suggesting a potential infection."
"The epidural analgesia was administered 6 hours ago for pain management."
"Oxytocin (Pitocin) was initiated 8 hours ago to augment labor progress."
"The patient's blood pressure is 130/80 mmHg, and her temperature is 37.5°C (99.5°F).

Ans 5:

"The fetal heart rate is monitored continuously, and it is within the normal range."

This statement is not indicative of a complication. Continuous monitoring of the fetal heart rate is a standard practice during labor to assess the well-being of the baby.

"Sarah's white blood cell count is elevated, suggesting a potential infection."

This statement is indicative of a potential complication. An elevated white blood cell count suggests the presence of an infection, which is a concerning factor during labor.

"The epidural analgesia was administered 6 hours ago for pain management."

This statement is indicative of a management intervention but does not directly point to a complication. However, the fact that Sarah is now experiencing increased pain suggests a change in her condition.

"Oxytocin (Pitocin) was initiated 8 hours ago to augment labor progress."

This statement is indicative of a management intervention. Oxytocin is commonly used to augment labor, but its initiation time is mentioned to provide a context of the ongoing labor process.
Incorrect Answer: "The patient's blood pressure is 130/80 mmHg, and her temperature is 37.5°C (99.5°F)."

This statement provides information about the patient's vital signs, but it does not directly indicate a complication. However, vital signs are essential to monitor for any changes that may signal distress.

Que 6: Prolonged labor in a primigravida, or a first-time mother, can present several challenges and requires careful management. One common challenge associated with prolonged labor is increased risk of _____ delivery.
A) vaginal
B) operative
C) spontaneous
D) elective

Answer: Prolonged labor in a primigravida, or a first-time mother, can present several challenges and requires careful management. One common challenge associated with prolonged labor is increased risk of **operative** delivery.

A) Vaginal:
- Vaginal delivery is the natural method of childbirth and does not specifically indicate a complication related to prolonged labor. Prolonged labor often necessitates interventions beyond normal vaginal delivery.

C) Spontaneous:
- Spontaneous delivery refers to childbirth that occurs naturally without medical intervention. However, prolonged labor usually requires medical interventions and monitoring, reducing the likelihood of a spontaneous delivery.

D) Elective:
- Elective delivery refers to a planned delivery, often scheduled in advance, which doesn't typically relate to complications from prolonged labor. Prolonged labor usually involves urgent or necessary interventions rather than elective ones.

B) Operative:
- **Correct Answer:** Prolonged labor can increase the risk of an operative delivery, such as a cesarean section or the use of forceps/vacuum extraction. These are necessary interventions when labor is not progressing as expected, ensuring the safety of both mother and baby.

CASE STUDY 4: Management Strategies for Paranoid Schizophrenia

Patient Information:

Name: Mr. John Doe
Age: 25 years
Gender: Male
Admission Date: 2023-12-15

Nurse's Notes:

History:
Mr. Doe is a 25-year-old male admitted with a diagnosis of paranoid schizophrenia. According to the patient's family, he has a history of behavioral changes, increasing social withdrawal, and auditory hallucinations over the past six months. No known family history of psychiatric disorders was reported.

Vital Signs:

Blood Pressure: 120/80 mmHg
Heart Rate: 80 bpm
Respiratory Rate: 18 breaths/min
Temperature: 98.6°F (37°C)
Oxygen Saturation: 98%

Medications:

Olanzapine 10 mg, oral, once daily: Administered at bedtime to manage positive symptoms and prevent relapse.
Lorazepam 2 mg, oral, PRN (as needed) for severe agitation: Used for crisis intervention during acute exacerbations.

Laboratory Results:

Complete Blood Count (CBC): Within normal limits.
Liver Function Tests (LFTs): Within normal limits.
Renal Function Tests (RFTs): Within normal limits.
Serum Olanzapine Level: Not checked (routine monitoring not indicated).

Que 1:

Which of the following behaviors of the patient is indicative of positive symptoms of schizophrenia?

Options:

A. Social withdrawal and lack of motivation

B. Auditory hallucinations and paranoid delusions

C. Flat affect and diminished emotional expression

D. Impaired memory and attention deficits

E. Excessive motor activity and catatonic behavior

F. Inability to initiate or complete activities of daily living

G. Hyperactivity and rapid speech patterns

Ans 1:

Correct Answers: B, E, G

Explanation:

A. Social withdrawal and lack of motivation: These are examples of negative symptoms of schizophrenia, not positive symptoms. Negative symptoms involve deficits in normal emotional and behavioral functioning.

B. Auditory hallucinations and paranoid delusions: These are classic examples of positive symptoms. Auditory hallucinations involve hearing voices, while paranoid delusions involve irrational beliefs of persecution or harm.

C. Flat affect and diminished emotional expression: These are also negative symptoms and do not reflect the presence of positive symptoms such as hallucinations or delusions.

D. Impaired memory and attention deficits: These are cognitive symptoms, which are a distinct category from positive symptoms. Cognitive symptoms may affect memory, attention, and executive functions.

E. Excessive motor activity and catatonic behavior: Excessive motor activity and catatonic behavior are examples of positive symptoms. Catatonia involves a range of motor behaviors, including stupor or excessive, purposeless motor activity.

F. Inability to initiate or complete activities of daily living: This is another example of negative symptoms, as it reflects a lack of motivation or ability to engage in typical daily activities.

G. Hyperactivity and rapid speech patterns: These are examples of positive symptoms. Hyperactivity and rapid speech can be indicative of agitation or thought disorders commonly seen in schizophrenia.

Que 2:

In the nursing care provided for Mr. Doe, which actions align with the principles of trauma-informed care and legal/ethical considerations?

Options:

A. Regularly involving the patient's family in decision-making processes.

B. Applying trauma-informed care principles to recognize potential trauma experiences.

C. Monitoring and documenting vital signs during acute phases.

D. Adhering to legal and ethical standards by ensuring involuntary hospitalization.

E. Collaborating with interprofessional teams for comprehensive care.

F. Emphasizing the importance of ongoing risk assessment for self-harm.

G. Maintaining accurate documentation for effective communication within the team.

Ans 2:

B. Applying trauma-informed care principles to recognize potential trauma experiences.
E. Collaborating with interprofessional teams for comprehensive care.
G. Maintaining accurate documentation for effective communication within the team.

Explanation:

- A. Regularly involving the patient's family in decision-making processes: While involving family can be beneficial, it may not always align with trauma-informed care if the family is a source of trauma. It depends on the patient's specific situation and preferences.

- B. Applying trauma-informed care principles to recognize potential trauma experiences: This is a key aspect of trauma-informed care, which focuses on understanding and addressing the impact of trauma on the patient.

- C. Monitoring and documenting vital signs during acute phases: This is important for overall patient care but does not specifically address trauma-informed care or legal/ethical considerations.

- D. Adhering to legal and ethical standards by ensuring involuntary hospitalization: While ensuring adherence to legal and ethical standards is important, involuntary hospitalization should be considered carefully and only when absolutely necessary. It may not always align with trauma-informed care principles, which emphasize patient autonomy and empowerment.

- E. Collaborating with interprofessional teams for comprehensive care: This aligns with both trauma-informed care and legal/ethical considerations, as it ensures that the patient receives holistic and well-coordinated care.

- F. Emphasizing the importance of ongoing risk assessment for self-harm: This is crucial for patient safety and aligns with legal/ethical considerations, but it is not specifically related to trauma-informed care principles.

- G. Maintaining accurate documentation for effective communication within the team: Accurate documentation is essential for legal/ethical considerations and ensures that all team members are informed about the patient's care.

Que 3:

Identify the correct rows

Symptom/Management Aspect	Description	Is this correct? (Yes/No)
Positive Symptoms	Hallucinations, delusions, thought disorders.	
Negative Symptoms	Social withdrawal, lack of motivation, diminished emotional expression.	
Cognitive Symptoms	Memory deficits, attention issues, executive function impairment.	
Antipsychotic Medications	Clozapine, risperidone, and olanzapine are commonly prescribed.	
Psychotherapy	Cognitive-behavioral therapy (CBT) helps cope with challenges.	
Crisis Intervention	Strategies for acute exacerbations to ensure patient and others' safety.	
Self-Care Promotion	Encouraging personal hygiene, nutrition, and engagement in meaningful activities.	
Involuntary Hospitalization	Commonly recommended for better long-term outcomes.	

Answer 3:

Symptom/Management Aspect	Description	Is this correct? (Yes/No)
Positive Symptoms	Hallucinations, delusions, thought disorders.	Yes
Negative Symptoms	Social withdrawal, lack of motivation, diminished emotional expression.	Yes
Cognitive Symptoms	Memory deficits, attention issues, executive function impairment.	Yes
Antipsychotic Medications	Clozapine, risperidone, and olanzapine are commonly prescribed.	Yes
Psychotherapy	Cognitive-behavioral therapy (CBT) helps cope with challenges.	Yes

Crisis Intervention	Strategies for acute exacerbations to ensure patient and others' safety.	Yes
Self-Care Promotion	Encouraging personal hygiene, nutrition, and engagement in meaningful activities.	Yes
Involuntary Hospitalization	Commonly recommended for better long-term outcomes.	No

Correct Rows Explanation:

Positive Symptoms: This row is correct. Positive symptoms in schizophrenia include hallucinations (perceptions without external stimuli), delusions (false beliefs), and thought disorders.

Cognitive Symptoms: This row is correct. Cognitive symptoms involve deficits in cognitive functions such as memory, attention, and executive functions. This is a distinct category of symptoms in schizophrenia.

Negative Symptoms: This row is incorrect. Negative symptoms of schizophrenia include social withdrawal, lack of motivation, and diminished emotional expression. In the table, it's marked as "No" to indicate that it's not a correct aspect related to positive symptoms.

Involuntary Hospitalization: This row is incorrect. Involuntary hospitalization is not commonly recommended for better long-term outcomes in schizophrenia. While it may be necessary in certain situations, it's generally considered a last resort due to ethical and legal considerations. In the table, it's marked as "No" to indicate that it's not a correct statement about the management of schizophrenia.

Que 4:

Read the following statements provided by a patient's caretaker and identify which sentences are related to schizophrenia. Explain why each statement is either right or wrong.

Statements:

1. "My loved one often talks about feeling persecuted and spied upon by unseen forces."
2. "They have been withdrawn and avoid social interactions lately, even with close family members."
3. "There's a noticeable decline in their ability to focus, and they seem to struggle with memory issues."
4. "We are considering enrolling them in a vocational rehabilitation program to improve job prospects."
5. "The doctor has prescribed antipsychotic medication to manage their symptoms."
6. "They exhibit hyperactivity and impulsive behavior at times, which is concerning."
7. "I've noticed that they have become increasingly interested in pursuing creative activities like painting."
8. "The family is actively involved in decision-making processes and the patient's recovery."
9. "The therapist recommended cognitive-behavioral therapy to help with coping skills."
10. "We are constantly monitoring for any signs of self-harm or harm to others, especially during acute phases."

Ans 4:

1. **"My loved one often talks about feeling persecuted and spied upon by unseen forces."**
   - **Related to Schizophrenia:** Yes
   - **Explanation:** This describes paranoid delusions, which are a common positive symptom of schizophrenia. Individuals may believe they are being persecuted or watched without evidence.

2. **"They have been withdrawn and avoid social interactions lately, even with close family members."**
   - **Related to Schizophrenia:** Yes
   - **Explanation:** Social withdrawal is a negative symptom of schizophrenia. It reflects a decline in social engagement and interest in relationships.

3. **"There's a noticeable decline in their ability to focus, and they seem to struggle with memory issues."**
   - **Related to Schizophrenia:** Yes
   - **Explanation:** Cognitive symptoms of schizophrenia include impaired attention, memory, and executive functioning.

4. **"We are considering enrolling them in a vocational rehabilitation program to improve job prospects."**
   - **Related to Schizophrenia:** No
   - **Explanation:** While vocational rehabilitation can benefit individuals with schizophrenia, this statement does not describe a symptom or behavior directly related to the condition.

5. **"The doctor has prescribed antipsychotic medication to manage their symptoms."**
   - **Related to Schizophrenia:** Yes
   - **Explanation:** Antipsychotic medications are commonly prescribed to manage the positive symptoms of schizophrenia, such as hallucinations and delusions.

6. **"They exhibit hyperactivity and impulsive behavior at times, which is concerning."**
   - **Related to Schizophrenia:** No
   - **Explanation:** Hyperactivity and impulsive behavior are not typical symptoms of schizophrenia. These symptoms are more characteristic of other conditions, such as ADHD or bipolar disorder.

7. **"I've noticed that they have become increasingly interested in pursuing creative activities like painting."**
   - **Related to Schizophrenia:** No
   - **Explanation:** An increased interest in creative activities is not specifically related to schizophrenia and could be a positive development in any individual's life.

8. **"The family is actively involved in decision-making processes and the patient's recovery."**
   - **Related to Schizophrenia:** No
   - **Explanation:** Family involvement is important in the care and recovery of individuals with schizophrenia, but the statement itself does not describe a symptom of the condition.

9. **"The therapist recommended cognitive-behavioral therapy to help with coping skills."**
   - **Related to Schizophrenia:** Yes
   - **Explanation:** Cognitive-behavioral therapy (CBT) is often used as part of the treatment plan for schizophrenia to help patients develop coping skills and manage symptoms.

10. **"We are constantly monitoring for any signs of self-harm or harm to others, especially during acute phases."**
    - **Related to Schizophrenia:** Yes
    - **Explanation:** Monitoring for self-harm or harm to others is important in schizophrenia, particularly during acute phases when symptoms may be more severe and risk factors for self-harm or aggression may be heightened.

Que 5:

Read the following and choose the right answers:

As we delve into understanding and managing schizophrenia, it becomes evident that the multifaceted nature of this mental health disorder requires comprehensive approaches. When it comes to the _____ (1. onset/etiology) of schizophrenia, the interplay of genetic, environmental, and neurobiological factors remains a complex puzzle. Individuals with schizophrenia may exhibit a range of symptoms, including positive, negative, and cognitive manifestations, each impacting their daily lives differently. In terms of treatment, a combination of medication, psychotherapy, and psychosocial support is often employed. The choice between _____ (2. antipsychotic/antidepressant) medications depends on the specific symptoms and needs of the individual. Similarly, the incorporation of therapeutic strategies such as cognitive-behavioral therapy (CBT) or supportive counseling plays a crucial role in fostering recovery. Whether considering the _____ (3. acute/chronic) nature of schizophrenia, early intervention remains pivotal for improved outcomes. Finally, as healthcare providers, maintaining _____ (4. cultural/ethical) competence in our approach ensures the delivery of patient-centered care that respects individual values and fosters a supportive environment.

Ans 5:

(1. onset/etiology): The correct answer is "etiology." Etiology refers to the study of the causes of a disease, which is more relevant to understanding the factors contributing to the development of schizophrenia. Onset, while related, specifically refers to the time when the symptoms first appear.

(2. antipsychotic/antidepressant): The correct answer is "antipsychotic." Antipsychotic medications are commonly prescribed for managing symptoms of schizophrenia, helping control positive symptoms such as hallucinations and delusions. Antidepressants are not typically the first line of treatment for schizophrenia.

(3. acute/chronic): The correct answer is "chronic." Schizophrenia is generally considered a chronic condition with persistent symptoms, although the severity may fluctuate over time. Acute refers more to the intensity of symptoms during certain phases.

(4. cultural/ethical): The correct answer is "cultural." While both cultural and ethical considerations are important in healthcare, the emphasis in the context of schizophrenia management is often on cultural competence. Understanding cultural factors helps tailor care to the individual's background and beliefs, fostering effective communication and collaboration in treatment.

Que 6:

Which of the following statements about medications used in the treatment of schizophrenia is correct?

Options:

A. Antidepressants are the primary medications prescribed for managing positive symptoms.

B. Antipsychotic medications, such as clozapine and risperidone, are commonly prescribed to manage symptoms.

C. Benzodiazepines are the first-line treatment for cognitive symptoms associated with schizophrenia.

D. Medication is generally not recommended as a part of schizophrenia treatment.

Ans 6:

Correct Answer: B

Explanation:

A. Antidepressants are the primary medications prescribed for managing positive symptoms: This statement is incorrect. Antidepressants are not the primary medications for managing positive symptoms of schizophrenia. Antipsychotic medications are the mainstay for addressing positive symptoms like hallucinations and delusions.

B. Antipsychotic medications, such as clozapine and risperidone, are commonly prescribed to manage symptoms: This statement is correct. Antipsychotic medications, including clozapine and risperidone, are commonly prescribed to manage both positive and, to some extent, negative symptoms of schizophrenia. They work by modulating neurotransmitter imbalances in the brain.

C. Benzodiazepines are the first-line treatment for cognitive symptoms associated with schizophrenia: This statement is incorrect. While benzodiazepines may be used in some cases to manage anxiety or agitation, they are not considered first-line treatment for cognitive symptoms. Cognitive symptoms are often addressed through other therapeutic interventions.

D. Medication is generally not recommended as a part of schizophrenia treatment: This statement is incorrect. Medication, particularly antipsychotic medications, is a fundamental component of schizophrenia treatment. These medications help manage symptoms and prevent relapses, playing a crucial role in the overall care of individuals with schizophrenia.

CASE STUDY 5: Effective Transfusion Management

Patient's History: Mark, a 45-year-old male, was admitted to the hospital due to severe bleeding from an injury. A diagnosis revealed a severe case of thrombocytopenia, necessitating an urgent blood transfusion.

Nurse's Observations:

During Mark's care, the nursing team took meticulous steps to ensure a safe and effective transfusion process:

Verified the patient's identification band and cross-checked it with the blood sample.

Ensured Rh and ABO compatibility of the blood sample before initiating transfusion.

Administered 1 unit of packed red blood cells (PRBCs) to boost erythrocytes for improved oxygen transport.

Transfused 2 units of platelets to address thrombocytopenia and enhance clotting.

Monitored vital signs throughout and after the transfusion.

Checked laboratory values for erythrocyte and platelet count 4-6 hours post-transfusion.

Medications Administered:

Packed Red Blood Cells (PRBCs):

Dosage: 1 unit

Platelets:

Dosage: 2 units

Lab Values:

Mark's response to the transfusion was evident in the improved laboratory values:

Hemoglobin: Increased from 8 g/dL to 9 g/dL.

Hematocrit: Rose from 24% to 27%.

Platelet Count: Increased from 50,000 to 150,000.

Que 1: Which of the following lab values indicates an improvement in the patient's clotting ability after the transfusion of 2 units of platelets?

A) Hemoglobin
B) Hematocrit

C) Platelet count
D) White blood cell count

Ans 1:

Answer: C) Platelet count

Explanation:
Platelets play a crucial role in clotting and preventing bleeding. A low platelet count increases the risk of bleeding and hampers clotting ability. The normal platelet range is typically between 150,000 and 450,000 platelets per microliter of blood. In this case, the patient initially had thrombocytopenia with a platelet count of 50,000 before the transfusion. After receiving 2 units of platelets, the count increased to 150,000, signifying an enhancement in clotting ability.

Additional Information:

Hemoglobin and Hematocrit: These values measure red blood cell levels and oxygen-carrying capacity, unrelated to clotting ability.
White Blood Cell Count: Reflects immune system function, not directly tied to clotting ability.

Que 2: Drag correct options to the blank spaces given:

Severe thrombocytopenia is a condition characterized by a _____ in platelet count, which can lead to an increased risk of _____. Nursing management for this condition may include which of the following interventions?

A) Encouraging the patient to participate in contact sports to increase activity levels
B) Administering aspirin to prevent blood clots
C) Implementing fall prevention measures
D) Encouraging the patient to take hot baths to improve circulation
E) Increase
F) Decrease

Ans 2:

Answer: F) Decrease and C) Implementing fall prevention measures

Explanation:

Severe thrombocytopenia is a condition in which there is a decrease in the number of platelets in the blood, which can lead to an increased risk of bleeding. The goal of nursing management in this case is to prevent bleeding complications by implementing measures to reduce the risk of injury. Hence first blank space should be filled by dragging option F.

For second space, Option A is incorrect because participating in contact sports can increase the risk of injury and further bleeding. Option B is incorrect because aspirin is an antiplatelet medication that can increase the risk of bleeding in patients with thrombocytopenia. Option D is incorrect because hot baths can cause blood vessels to dilate and increase the risk of bleeding. Therefore, the correct answer is C) Implementing fall prevention measures, which may include removing obstacles from the patient's environment, using bed rails or other restraints, and encouraging the patient to use assistive devices such as a walker or cane. These measures can help prevent falls and other injuries that could result in bleeding complications in patients with thrombocytopenia.

Que 3: Which of the following is the primary purpose of transfusing packed red blood cells in this case?

A) To address thrombocytopenia
B) To increase hemoglobin and hematocrit levels
C) To improve clotting
D) To provide additional white blood cells

Ans 3:

Answer: B) To increase hemoglobin and hematocrit levels

Explanation:

The nurse's notes indicate that the patient was transfused with 1 unit of packed red blood cells, which are used to increase the erythrocytes for oxygen transportation. Hemoglobin and hematocrit are both measures of the amount of red blood cells present in the blood. Hemoglobin is the protein in red blood cells that carries oxygen throughout the body, while hematocrit is the percentage of red blood cells in the total volume of blood. By increasing the number of red blood cells, the transfusion aims to increase the patient's oxygen-carrying capacity, which is particularly important in cases of anemia. The increase in hemoglobin and hematocrit levels after the transfusion indicates that the transfusion was successful in achieving this goal. Therefore, the correct answer is B) To increase hemoglobin and hematocrit levels.

Que 4: What was the outcome of Mark's blood transfusion in the hospital?

A) Hemoglobin and hematocrit both decreased after the transfusion.
B) Hemoglobin and hematocrit both increased after the transfusion.
C) Hemoglobin decreased and hematocrit increased after the transfusion.
D) Hemoglobin increased and hematocrit decreased after the transfusion.
E) There was no change in hemoglobin and hematocrit after the transfusion.
F) The transfusion was not successful and the patient's vital signs were not monitored.
G) The transfusion was not successful and the blood sample was not checked for compatibility.

Ans 4:
Correct Options: B

Explanation:
- Option B is correct as per the lab values, hemoglobin increased from 8 g/dL to 9 g/dL and hematocrit increased from 24% to 27% after the transfusion.
- Option F is incorrect as per the nurse's notes, the patient's vital signs were monitored during and after the transfusion.
- Option A, C, D, E, and G are incorrect as they are not supported by the patient's history and nurse's notes.

Que 5: What is the correct procedure for blood transfusion in patient with severe thrombocytopenia?

A) Transfuse 2 units of packed red blood cells and 1 unit of platelets
B) Transfuse 1 unit of packed red blood cells and 2 units of platelets
C) Transfuse 2 units of red blood cells and no platelets
D) Transfuse 1 unit of red blood cells and no platelets

Ans 5:

Answer: B) Transfuse 1 unit of packed red blood cells and 2 units of platelets

Explanation:
A) Transfusing 2 units of packed red blood cells would not address the thrombocytopenia and would not improve the patient's clotting. The patient's hematocrit only increased from 24% to 27% after transfusing 1 unit of packed red blood cells.
B) This option is correct as per the physician's order, the nurse's notes and the lab values after the transfusion. 1 unit of packed red blood cells was transfused to increase the erythrocytes for oxygen transportation and 2 units of platelets were transfused to address the thrombocytopenia and improve clotting. The laboratory values showed an increase in hematocrit and platelet count after the transfusion.
C) Transfusing 2 units of red blood cells without platelets would not address the thrombocytopenia and would not improve the patient's clotting. The patient was diagnosed with a severe case of thrombocytopenia and required platelets for improvement.
D) Transfusing 1 unit of red blood cells without platelets would increase the erythrocytes for oxygen transportation but would not address the thrombocytopenia and would not improve the patient's clotting. The patient was diagnosed with a severe case of thrombocytopenia and required platelets for improvement.

Que 6: Which of the following nursing procedures is a critical step in ensuring patient safety during blood transfusion?

A) Verifying the patient's identity and blood product compatibility at the bedside using two unique identifiers
B) Administering antipyretics routinely before starting the transfusion to prevent febrile reactions
C) Infusing the blood product as quickly as possible to minimize the risk of contamination
D) Using a standard IV solution like dextrose to dilute the blood product before administration

Ans: A
Explanation:

A) Verifying the patient's identity and blood product compatibility at the bedside using two unique identifiers

This is a critical step in ensuring patient safety during blood transfusions. Proper identification of the patient and cross-checking the blood product against the patient's records helps prevent potentially fatal errors, such as transfusion reactions due to ABO incompatibility.

B) Administering antipyretics routinely before starting the transfusion to prevent febrile reactions

While antipyretics (e.g., acetaminophen) may be given prophylactically in some cases to reduce the risk of febrile non-hemolytic transfusion reactions, this is not considered a universal or critical step. It is more of a supportive measure and not essential for ensuring safety.

C) Infusing the blood product as quickly as possible to minimize the risk of contamination

Blood products should be infused at a controlled rate to prevent complications such as fluid overload or acute transfusion reactions. Rapid infusion can be dangerous and is not recommended unless specifically indicated (e.g., massive hemorrhage). Additionally, blood products must be used within 4 hours of issuance from the blood bank, but speed is not the priority.

D) Using a standard IV solution like dextrose to dilute the blood product before administration

Blood products should never be diluted with dextrose or other IV solutions, as this can cause hemolysis of red blood cells. Only normal saline (0.9% sodium chloride) is compatible with blood products.

CASE STUDY 6: Management of Electrolyte Imbalance

Patient's History: Mr. John, a 65-year-old male, was admitted to the hospital with complaints of confusion, muscle weakness, and seizures. His past medical history was significant for high blood pressure and diabetes. He was on diuretic medications for the past few months. On examination, his blood pressure was found to be low and his pulse was weak.

Nurse's Notes: 1/31, Admitted with complaints of confusion, muscle weakness, and seizures.

BP: 90/60 mmHg, Pulse: weak PMH: HTN, DM On diuretic meds 2/1, Sodium level: 125 mEq/L (Hyponatremia) Started on sodium chloride IV infusions. Potassium level: 3.2 mEq/L (Hypokalemia)

Medications:

Sodium Chloride IV Infusion:

Dose: Dosage administered based on the physician's order.

Diuretic Medication Adjustment:

Dose: Dosage adjusted as per physician's order.

Lab Values: Sodium: 125 mEq/L Potassium: 3.2 mEq/L

Que 1: What is the most likely cause of the patient's confusion, muscle weakness, and seizures?

A) Hypertension
B) Diabetes Mellitus
C) Hyponatremia
D) Hypokalemia
E) Diuretic medication

Ans 1:

Correct Options: C) Hyponatremia and D) Hypokalemia

Explanation:
- Hyponatremia (low sodium levels) is noted in the patient's lab values (125 mEq/L). Symptoms of hyponatremia include confusion, muscle weakness, and seizures, which are also present in the patient.
- Hypokalemia (low potassium levels) is also noted in the patient's lab values (3.2 mEq/L) and can cause similar symptoms. Hypokalemia (low potassium levels) can cause muscle weakness, cramps, arrhythmias, and fatigue, but it does not typically cause seizures or confusion. The neurological symptoms described here are more characteristic of hyponatremia.

- HTN and DM are present in the patient's PMH (past medical history), but are not the immediate cause of the symptoms.

- The diuretic medication the patient was on may have contributed to the low electrolyte levels. However, the main cause is the low sodium and potassium levels.

Que 2. What is the most likely cause of the patient's hyponatremia and hypokalemia?

A. Excessive fluid intake
B. Increased use of diuretics
C. Kidney disease
D. Medication side effect

Ans 2:

Answer: B. Increased use of diuretics

Explanation:
- The patient is admitted with symptoms of confusion, muscle weakness, and seizures and has a low blood pressure and weak pulse.
- The patient has a history of hypertension and diabetes and is on diuretic medication.
- The sodium level is low (125 mEq/L) and the potassium level is also low (3.2 mEq/L).
- The physician has ordered a reduction in the dose of diuretic medication and a dietary restriction of sodium.

These factors suggest that the increased use of diuretics is the most likely cause of the patient's hyponatremia and hypokalemia. Option A (excessive fluid intake) is not likely since the patient has a low blood pressure and is being monitored for electrolyte levels. Option C (kidney disease) may also contribute, but the focus is on reducing the dose of diuretics and dietary restrictions of sodium. Option D (medication side effect) is also a possibility, but the focus is on the patient's use of diuretics.

Que 3. What is the correct nursing intervention for the patient with hyponatremia and hypokalemia as noted in the scenario?

A) Stop sodium chloride IV infusion
B) Increase dose of diuretic medication
C) No dietary restriction of sodium
D) Monitor fluid intake and output

Ans 3:

Correct Option: D) Monitor fluid intake and output

Explanation: A) Stopping the sodium chloride IV infusion would be detrimental to the patient as they are suffering from hyponatremia, which is a low level of sodium in the blood. Sodium chloride infusion is necessary to replenish the sodium levels.
B) Increasing the dose of diuretic medication would further lower the potassium levels, as diuretics increase urine output and can result in the loss of potassium and other electrolytes.
C) No dietary restriction of sodium would not be appropriate as the patient is already suffering from hyponatremia, which could be due to excessive sodium intake. The dietary restriction of sodium is necessary to regulate sodium levels.
D) Monitoring fluid intake and output is important to ensure that the patient is not retaining excess fluid and electrolytes. This will help to regulate the electrolyte levels and prevent further fluctuations.

Que 4: What nursing intervention should be taken for the patient's electrolyte imbalances?

A. Increase the dose of diuretic medication
B. Stop sodium chloride IV infusions
C. Remove dietary restriction of sodium
D. Monitor electrolyte levels

Ans 4:

Correct Answer: D. Monitor electrolyte levels

Explanation: The physician has already ordered the appropriate interventions for the patient's electrolyte imbalances including sodium chloride IV infusion, reducing the dose of diuretic medication, and dietary restriction of sodium. The most important intervention at this point is to monitor the patient's electrolyte levels to ensure they are improving and within normal range.
Option A is incorrect because increasing the dose of diuretic medication may worsen the patient's hyponatremia and hypokalemia.
Option B is incorrect because stopping the sodium chloride IV infusions may result in further decline of the patient's sodium levels.
Option C is incorrect because removing the dietary restriction of sodium may lead to further imbalances in the patient's electrolyte levels.

Que 5. What is the nursing intervention for Hyponatremia?

A. Provide sodium chloride IV infusions
B. Provide osmotic diuretics
C. Choose hormone replacement procedure
D. Reduce the dose of diuretics

Ans 5:

Correct option: A. Provide sodium chloride IV infusions

Explanation: If Hyponatremia is due to fluid or blood loss, vomiting or diarrhea, the nursing intervention would be to provide sodium chloride IV infusions. Option B is not correct as osmotic diuretics are used in case of excess fluid volume and not in case of Hyponatremia. Option C is incorrect as it is only applicable if the cause is Addison's disease. Option D is correct only if the cause of Hyponatremia is due to certain medications such as diuretics.

Que 6. What is the nursing intervention for hypokalemia?

A) Provide sodium chloride IV infusions
B) Administer diuretics
C) Supplement dietary potassium sources
D) Reduce the dose of drugs causing hypokalemia

Ans 6:

Correct Option: C) Supplement dietary potassium sources

Explanation: Option A) is incorrect as hypokalemia is not caused by fluid or blood loss and does not require sodium chloride IV infusions.

Option B) is incorrect as the use of diuretics may further deplete potassium levels.

Option D) is incorrect as reducing the dose of drugs causing hypokalemia may not be enough to treat the condition and may require additional interventions.

Option C) is correct as supplementing dietary potassium sources such as bananas, spinach, or other green leafy vegetables can help to raise potassium levels in cases of moderately low potassium levels. However, severe hypokalemic states may require supplemental potassium.

CASE STUDY 7: Management of Acute Exacerbation of Asthma

History and Nurse's Notes:
A 65-year-old male patient is admitted with symptoms of shortness of breath, cough, and wheezing. The patient has a history of smoking and asthma.

Nurse's Observations:

- Observed shortness of breath and wheezing during breathing.
- Chest sounds congested with wheezing and crackles.
- Elevated pulse rate at 120 bpm.
- Blood pressure measures 90/60 mmHg.
- Oxygen saturation recorded at 88% on room air.

2. Vital Signs:

- Pulse Rate: 120 bpm
- Blood Pressure: 90/60 mmHg
- Oxygen Saturation: 88%

3. Medications:

Prescribed Medications:

- Nebulization: For relief of wheezing and shortness of breath.

    Dosage: Administer 1 nebulization every 4 hours.

- Bronchodilators: To open up airways.

    Dosage: Take 2 puffs every 6 hours.

4. Lab Values:

ABG Test Results:

pH: 7.25

PaCO2: 50 mm Hg

HCO3: 20 mEq/L

O2 Sat: 88%

Que 1. What condition does the patient have based on the ABG test results?

A) Respiratory Acidosis
B) Respiratory Alkalosis
C) Metabolic Acidosis
D) Metabolic Alkalosis

Ans 1:

Answer: A) Respiratory Acidosis

Explanation: The patient's ABG test results show a low pH of 7.25, which indicates acidosis. The elevated PaCO2 of 50 mm Hg suggests that the acidosis is caused by decreased ventilation. The bicarbonate levels are below the normal range, which shows that the body is compensating for the acidosis. The oxygen saturation is also below normal, supporting the respiratory acidosis diagnosis. The patient's history of smoking and asthma further supports the diagnosis.

Que 2. What is the most likely diagnosis for the 65-year-old male patient based on the given information?

A) Chronic Obstructive Pulmonary Disease (COPD)
B) Bronchitis
C) Pneumonia
D) Acute Respiratory Distress Syndrome (ARDS)
E) Asthma exacerbation

Ans 2:

Answer: A) Chronic Obstructive Pulmonary Disease (COPD) and E) Asthma exacerbation are the correct answers.

Explanation: A) Chronic Obstructive Pulmonary Disease (COPD) is a likely diagnosis based on the patient's history of smoking and asthma, symptoms of shortness of breath, wheezing, and cough, chest sounds congested with wheezing and crackles, and elevated pulse rate.
B) Bronchitis is not a likely diagnosis as the patient's symptoms, such as shortness of breath, elevated pulse rate, and low blood pressure, suggest a more severe condition than just bronchitis.
C) Pneumonia is not a likely diagnosis as the patient's chest sounds congested with wheezing and crackles, which is not a typical sign of pneumonia.
D) Acute Respiratory Distress Syndrome (ARDS) is not a likely diagnosis as the patient's ABG results (pH 7.25 and PaCO2 50 mm Hg) do not meet the criteria for ARDS.
E) Asthma exacerbation is a correct answer as the patient has a history of asthma and is showing symptoms of wheezing and shortness of breath. The physician's order of nebulization and bronchodilators also supports this diagnosis.

Que 3. What is the primary cause of respiratory acidosis?

A) Hypoventilation
B) Pneumonia
C) Brain Trauma
D) Emphysema

Answer 3:
A) Hypoventilation

Explanation: Respiratory acidosis is caused by hypoventilation, which is when the lungs cannot exchange CO2 with the environment due to airway or ventilation obstruction. This causes the excess CO2 to combine with water to form carbonic acid, leading to an increase in hydrogen ions in the blood and a drop in the pH level. Other conditions such as pneumonia, brain trauma, and emphysema can also cause respiratory acidosis, but hypoventilation is the primary cause.

Que 4. What are the clinical manifestations of respiratory acidosis?

A. Seizures, warm and flushed skin, and decreased blood pressure
B. Drowsy and dizzy, headache, and coma
C. Tetany, numbness, and seizures
D. Deep and rapid respiration

Answer 4:

B. Drowsy and dizzy, headache, and coma

Explanation: The clinical manifestations of respiratory acidosis are related to the increase of carbonic acid in the blood, leading to hypoventilation. The compensatory mechanism of the kidneys retaining bicarbonate and excreting excess hydrogen ion can cause the patient to feel drowsy and dizzy, have a headache, and even go into a coma. Seizures, warm and flushed skin, and decreased blood pressure are also symptoms, but not specific to respiratory acidosis. Tetany, numbness, and seizures are the symptoms of respiratory alkalosis. Deep and rapid respiration is the symptom of metabolic acidosis.

Que 5. What is the main cause of metabolic alkalosis?

A. Excessive diarrhea
B. Diabetic ketoacidosis
C. Excessive vomiting
D. Kidney disease

Ans 5:

The main cause of metabolic alkalosis is C. Excessive vomiting. This occurs due to the loss of acid through increased bicarbonate ion concentration in the blood. Other causes include diuretics and citrate toxicity during massive transfusion of whole blood.

Que 6: What is the condition caused by excessive vomiting that leads to increase in bicarbonate ion concentration in blood?

A) Respiratory Alkalosis
B) Respiratory Acidosis
C) Metabolic Acidosis
D) Metabolic Alkalosis

Ans 6:

D) Metabolic Alkalosis

Explanation: Metabolic alkalosis is the condition caused by excessive vomiting that leads to increase in bicarbonate ion concentration in blood. This increase in bicarbonate ion concentration leads to loss of acid in the blood and results in metabolic alkalosis. Other causes of metabolic alkalosis include diuretics and citrate toxicity during massive transfusion of whole blood.

CASE STUDY 8: Management and Treatment Strategies for Burn Injuries

Patient's History Case Study: A 35-year-old male was admitted to the hospital with burn injuries on his left arm and leg caused by a chemical substance. He was brought to the emergency room within an hour of the injury. The patient reported a tingling sensation on the affected area and his skin appeared to be red on the surface and white on deeper areas.

Nurse's Notes:
- Started supplemental oxygen and monitored the patient's respiratory status closely.
- Assessed the patient's airways, breathing, and circulation (ABCs) and found them to be stable.
- Assessed the fluid loss and started fluid resuscitation using the Modified Brooke formula.
- Monitored the patient's urinary output and peripheral pulses.
- Kept the patient warm and removed all the clothes from the affected part.
- Started cardiac monitoring and assessed the patient's neurologic status, including consciousness and pain.
- Documented the patient's vital signs and fluid intake and output regularly.

Physician's Order:
- Administer supplemental oxygen as needed.
- Start fluid resuscitation using the Modified Brooke formula.
- Monitor the patient's respiratory status, urinary output, and peripheral pulses.
- Keep the patient warm and remove all the clothes from the affected part.
- Start cardiac monitoring and assess the patient's neurologic status regularly.
- Provide balanced restorative diet and drinks for nutritional support.
- Monitor the patient's vitals signs and fluid intake and output regularly.
- Focus on infection control, pain management, and physical therapy during the acute phase.

Lab Values:
- Hemoglobin: 12.5 g/dL
- White Blood Cell Count: 8,500/mm3
- Sodium: 137 mEq/L
- Potassium: 4.5 mEq/L
- Chloride: 102 mEq/L
- Bicarbonate: 24 mEq/L

Que 1. What is the most important priority for the patient in the scenario described above?

- A) Infection control
- B) Pain management
- C) Physical therapy
- D) Fluid resuscitation

Ans 1:

Answer: D) Fluid resuscitation

Explanation: A) Infection control is important, but it is not the most pressing priority in this scenario. The patient has just suffered burn injuries and is at high risk of fluid loss, dehydration, and electrolyte imbalances, making fluid resuscitation the top priority.
B) Pain management is also important, but it should not be prioritized above fluid resuscitation in this scenario.
C) Physical therapy is important for the patient's recovery, but it is not the most pressing priority in this acute phase.
D) Fluid resuscitation using the Modified Brooke formula is the most important priority as the patient has suffered burn injuries and is at high risk of fluid loss and dehydration. The patient's hemoglobin levels, white blood cell count, sodium, potassium, chloride, and bicarbonate levels are all indicators of the need for fluid resuscitation.

Que 2: Which formula is used for fluid resuscitation in the patient with burn injuries?

A) Modified Parkland
B) Modified Brooke
C) Parkland
D) Ringer's lactate

Answer 2:

C) Parkland Formula

Explanation: The Parkland Formula is widely used to calculate the amount of fluid required for burn patients over a 24-hour period. It helps guide the administration of intravenous fluids to ensure adequate resuscitation and prevent complications such as burn shock.

Que 2. What is the goal of the Acute phase in the management of burns?

A) To restore the patient's fluid levels
B) To restore the patient's condition to normal until wound closure is achieved
C) To focus on wound care and pain control
D) To monitor the patient's vital signs
E) To check the patient's peripheral pulses
F) To monitor the fluid intake and output
G) To monitor the patient's cardiac rhythm
H) To focus on infection control, pain management and physical therapy

Ans 2:
H) To focus on infection control, pain management, and physical therapy

Explanation: The Acute phase in the management of burns involves several crucial goals, including:
1. **Infection Control:** Preventing infection is a top priority due to the high risk associated with burn injuries.
2. **Pain Management:** Effective pain control is essential for patient comfort and recovery.
3. **Physical Therapy:** Early physical therapy helps in maintaining mobility, preventing contractures, and promoting healing.

While the other options (A, B, C, D, E, F, G) are important aspects of burn management, they may not encompass the comprehensive goals specifically associated with the Acute phase, which focuses on infection control, pain management, and physical therapy.

Que 3. Which of the following types of burns are not requiring skin grafting?

A. Superficial thickness burns
B. Superficial partial-thickness burns
C. Deep partial-thickness burns
D. Full-thickness burns
E. Deep full-thickness burns

Answer 3:
A. Superficial thickness burns

Explanation: Superficial thickness burns, also known as first-degree burns, affect only the outer layer of the skin (epidermis) and typically heal without the need for skin grafting. These burns usually heal within 7 to 10 days and do not result in scarring1
B. Superficial partial-thickness burns can also heal on their own without the need for skin grafting, although skin grafting can be used for early healing.
C. Deep partial-thickness burns can require skin grafting if necessary.
D. Full-thickness burns always require skin grafting as the entire dermis and epidermis is destroyed.
E. Deep full-thickness burns can require skin grafting and also affect internal bones, muscles, and tissues.

Que 4. Which of the following is not a part of the resuscitative phase in the management of burns?
A. Assessment of airways, breathing, and circulation (ABCs)
B. Administering supplemental oxygen
C. Monitoring fluid intake and output
D. Monitoring cardiac rhythm
E. Monitoring pulmonary function
F. Giving balanced restorative diet and drinks
G. Focusing on infection control
H. Starting physical therapy

Ans 4:
H. Starting physical therapy
- Incorrect (not part of resuscitative phase).
  Physical therapy is not initiated during the resuscitative phase because the patient is often too unstable. Physical therapy becomes important during the acute phase (to prevent complications like contractures) and the rehabilitation phase (to restore function).

Que 5. What are the different phases of burn injury management and what are the goals of each phase?

A. Emergency phase - To provide basic first aid procedures and prevent hypovolemic shock.
B. Resuscitative phase - To restore the patient's condition to normal and provide wound care.
C. Acute phase - To monitor vitals, focus on wound care and pain control, and provide nutritional support.
D. Rehabilitative phase - To make the patient ready for self-care and gain normal function.
E. Assessment phase - To assess the patient's airways, breathing, and circulation.
F. Fluid replacement phase - To replace fluids until the patient returns to normal levels.
G. Pain management phase - To manage pain and provide physical therapy.
H. Infection control phase - To prevent infections and monitor the patient's pulmonary function.

Ans 5:

Explanation: A, C, and D are correct.

The emergency phase focuses on providing basic first aid procedures to prevent hypovolemic shock. The resuscitative phase focuses on restoring the patient's condition to normal and providing wound care. The acute phase focuses on monitoring vitals, focusing on wound care and pain control, and providing nutritional support. The rehabilitative phase focuses on making the patient ready for self-care and gaining normal function.
B is incorrect as the resuscitative phase is not the goal but a phase that focuses on restoring the patient's condition to normal and providing wound care.
E is incorrect as the assessment phase is part of the emergency phase but not a separate phase.
F is incorrect as the fluid replacement phase is a part of the resuscitative phase.
G is incorrect as the pain management phase is part of the acute phase.
H is incorrect as the infection control phase is part of the acute phase.

CASE STUDY 9: Managing Epilepsy

Patient's history case study: A 23-year-old female patient presents with a history of generalized seizures. The patient reports having absence seizures, which typically last a few seconds and cause her to appear daydreaming. The patient has also had tonic-clonic seizures in the past, characterized by muscle stiffness, loss of consciousness, and jerking of the limbs. The patient has a family history of epilepsy and has been diagnosed with a genetic disorder.

Nurse's notes:
- Patient presents with a history of generalized seizures, including absence and tonic-clonic seizures
- Patient appears to have a genetic disorder causing seizures
- Patient reports absence seizures last a few seconds and cause her to appear daydreaming
- Patient reports tonic-clonic seizures characterized by muscle stiffness, loss of consciousness, and jerking of the limbs

Medications-
Phenytoin:
Dosage: Administered as per physician's order.
Therapeutic Range: 10-20 mcg/mL
Current Level: 10 mcg/mL

Patient's Vital Signs:
Pulse Rate: 80 bpm
Blood Pressure: 120/80 mmHg
Respiratory Rate: 16 breaths per minute
Temperature: 98.6°F

Lab values:
- Phenytoin level: 10 mcg/mL (therapeutic range: 10-20 mcg/mL)

Que 1. What are the primary reasons for administering phenytoin to the patient in this case study?

A) To control the symptoms of the patient's genetic disorder
B) To treat the patient's absence seizures
C) To prevent tonic-clonic seizures
D) To reduce the patient's risk of developing side effects
E) To maintain good oral hygiene
F) To prevent interference with medication absorption
G) To ensure the effectiveness of birth control pills
H) To monitor for changes in the patient's lab values

Ans 1:

A) To control the symptoms of the patient's genetic disorder
- Incorrect.
  Phenytoin is not typically used to manage symptoms of genetic disorders unless those symptoms specifically involve seizures. This option is too vague and does not directly relate to phenytoin's mechanism of action.

B) To treat the patient's absence seizures
- Incorrect.
  Phenytoin is **not effective** for treating **absence seizures** (also called petit mal seizures). Absence seizures are typically managed with medications like ethosuximide, valproate, or lamotrigine. Phenytoin is ineffective because it targets different types of seizure activity.

C) To prevent tonic-clonic seizures
- Correct.
  Phenytoin is highly effective in preventing **tonic-clonic seizures** (formerly called grand mal seizures), which involve loss of consciousness, muscle rigidity, and convulsions. This is one of the primary indications for phenytoin use.

D) To reduce the patient's risk of developing side effects
- Incorrect.
  While managing side effects is important in any medication regimen, this is not a reason for administering phenytoin. Side effects (e.g., gingival hyperplasia, dizziness, rash) are a concern but do not justify its use.

E) To maintain good oral hygiene
- Incorrect.
  Gingival hyperplasia (overgrowth of gum tissue) is a known side effect of phenytoin. Maintaining good oral hygiene is important to minimize this complication, but it is not a reason for administering the drug.

F) To prevent interference with medication absorption
- Incorrect.
  This option refers to considerations for administering phenytoin (e.g., avoiding enteral feedings that may interfere with absorption). However, it is not a reason for prescribing the medication.

G) To ensure the effectiveness of birth control pills

- **Incorrect.**
  Phenytoin can reduce the effectiveness of hormonal contraceptives by inducing liver enzymes that increase their metabolism. While this interaction must be monitored, it is not a reason for administering phenytoin.

H) To monitor for changes in the patient's lab values
- **Incorrect.**
  Monitoring lab values (e.g., serum phenytoin levels, liver function tests) is essential to ensure therapeutic dosing and avoid toxicity. However, this is part of ongoing management, not a reason for prescribing the drug.

Que 2. What is the diagnosis of the 23-year-old female patient based on the given scenario?

A) Migraine
B) Epilepsy
C) Multiple sclerosis
D) Parkinson's disease
E) Depression
F) Stroke
G) Alzheimer's disease
H) Huntington's disease

Ans 2:

A) Migraine - Incorrect. Migraine is a type of headache, not a seizure disorder.
B) Epilepsy - Correct. The patient presents with a history of generalized seizures, including absence and tonic-clonic seizures and has a family history of epilepsy.
C) Multiple sclerosis - Incorrect. Multiple sclerosis is a disease of the central nervous system, not a seizure disorder.
D) Parkinson's disease - Incorrect. Parkinson's disease is a movement disorder, not a seizure disorder.
E) Depression - Incorrect. Depression is a mental health condition, not a seizure disorder.
F) Stroke - Incorrect. Stroke is a sudden loss of blood flow to the brain, not a seizure disorder.
G) Alzheimer's disease - Incorrect. Alzheimer's disease is a progressive brain disorder, not a seizure disorder.
H) Huntington's disease - Incorrect. Huntington's disease is a genetic disorder causing the progressive breakdown of nerve cells in the brain, not a seizure disorder.

Que 3. Which of the following is a type of generalized seizure?

A. Absence seizure
B. Simple partial seizure
C. Tonic clonic seizure
D. Atonic seizure

Ans 3:

The types of generalized seizures from the provided options are:
A. Absence seizure C. Tonic clonic seizure D. Atonic seizure

Explanation:
- **Absence seizure:** A type of generalized seizure characterized by brief, sudden lapses in attention and activity, often described as "staring spells."
- **Tonic clonic seizure:** A type of generalized seizure that involves both tonic (stiffening) and clonic (jerking) phases. It is also known as a grand mal seizure.
- **Atonic seizure:** A type of generalized seizure that involves a sudden loss of muscle tone, leading to a collapse or fall.

B. Simple partial seizure: This is not a type of generalized seizure. Instead, it is a type of focal (or partial) seizure that affects a specific area of the brain without loss of consciousness.

Que 4. Which of the following is not a nursing intervention for a patient taking phenytoin for seizure control?

A. Instructing the patient to take good care of oral hygiene
B. Relying on birth control pills for family planning
C. Avoiding the use of phenytoin during pregnancy
D. Administering antipsychotics and anti-coagulants with phenytoin

Ans 4:

Correct answer: D. Administering antipsychotics and anti-coagulants with phenytoin

Explanation: A. Instructing the patient to take good care of oral hygiene is a correct intervention as phenytoin can cause swelling and bleeding of the gums. B. Relying on birth control pills for family planning is incorrect as phenytoin can decrease the efficiency of birth control pills. C. Avoiding the use of phenytoin during pregnancy is correct as it is a category D medication and may cause harm to the growing fetus. D. Administering antipsychotics and anti-coagulants with phenytoin is incorrect as these medications may cause medical interaction with phenytoin and should be used with care or continuously monitored.

Que 5. What is the nursing intervention for a patient taking Phenytoin for their seizures?

A) Administering an anti-inflammatory medication to reduce swelling of gums
B) Discontinuing birth control pills as they are no longer effective
C) Instructing the patient to practice good oral hygiene to prevent bleeding gums
D) Increasing the dose of Phenytoin to reduce dizziness

Ans 5:

Correct Option: C) Instructing the patient to practice good oral hygiene to prevent bleeding gums

Explanation: Phenytoin is an antiseizure drug used to treat tonic clonic and partial seizures. One of its side effects is bleeding of gums, so the nurse should instruct the patient to take good care of their oral hygiene to prevent this.
Option A is incorrect as anti-inflammatory medication will not help with bleeding gums.
Option B is correct as Phenytoin can decrease the efficiency of birth control pills.
Option D is incorrect as increasing the dose of Phenytoin may worsen its side effects.

Que 6. Which is the correct statement about epilepsy or a seizure?

A. Epilepsy is a type of seizure

B. Seizure is a temporary malfunction of the brain caused by excessive electrical discharge
C. Tonic clonic seizures are caused by genetic or metabolic disorders
D. Epilepsy is caused by abnormal electrical activity in only one cerebral hemisphere

Ans 6:

Answer: B
Explanation: Seizure is a temporary malfunction of the brain caused by abnormal and excessive electrical discharge in the brain. This is the definition of epilepsy or a seizure.
Option A is incorrect as epilepsy is not a type of seizure but rather a condition characterized by repeated seizures.
Option C is correct as tonic clonic seizures are caused by genetic or metabolic disorders, however, it is not the definition of epilepsy or a seizure.
Option D is incorrect as in a generalized seizure, the abnormal electrical activity involves both cerebral hemispheres.

CASE STUDY 10: Prevention and Management Strategies for Pressure Ulcers

Patient's History: A 65-year-old male patient was admitted to the hospital with a history of pressure ulcers. The patient has been bedridden for the past 3 months and has a history of immobility. The patient has stage 3 pressure ulcers on his sacral and heel regions.

Nurse's Notes:
- Patient's skin is intact and warm to touch
- Patient's sacral and heel regions have visible ulcers with a sunken appearance and some visible body fat and serum
- Patient's sacral and heel regions are painful to touch
- Patient's mobility is limited, and he requires assistance to change positions

Vital Signs:

Blood Pressure: 120/80 mmHg
Pulse Rate: 72 beats per minute
Respiratory Rate: 16 breaths per minute
Temperature: 98.6°F (37°C)

Medication:
- Name: Acetaminophen
- Dosage: Administered as needed, following the physician's prescription guidelines.

Lab Values:
- WBC count: 8,000/mm3 (normal range: 4,500-11,000/mm3)
- Hb: 12 g/dL (normal range: 13.5-17.5 g/dL)
- Platelet count: 200,000/mm3 (normal range: 150,000-450,000/mm3)

Que 1: Which nursing intervention is appropriate for managing a patient with pressure ulcers as per the given nurse's notes and physician's order?

A. Administer antibiotics as needed
B. Apply honey dressing to the ulcers
C. Reposition the patient every 4 hours
D. Apply dressing to the sacral ulcer and calcium alginate gauze to the heel ulcer

Ans 1:

The correct answer is D. Apply dressing to the sacral ulcer and calcium alginate gauze to the heel ulcer. The nurse's notes indicate that the patient has pressure ulcers on the sacral and heel regions, and the physician's order instructs to clean and dress the ulcers daily, apply dressing to the sacral ulcer, and calcium alginate gauze to the heel ulcer. These interventions are important to promote healing, prevent infection, and reduce pain. Antibiotics may be administered if there is an infection, but it is not the first-line intervention. Honey dressing may have antimicrobial properties but is not mentioned in the physician's order. Repositioning the patient every 2 hours, as stated in the physician's order, helps to relieve pressure and prevent further damage to the skin. Option C, repositioning every 4 hours, is not an appropriate intervention for managing pressure ulcers.

Que 2. What type of dressing should be applied to the patient's stage 3 pressure ulcer on the sacral region?

A) Nontransparent hydrocolloid dressing
B) Composite film hydrocolloid dressing and hydrogels
C) Hydrocolloid hydrogel with foam dressing gauze
D) Calcium alginate gauze

Answer 2:
C) Hydrocolloid hydrogel with foam dressing gauze

Explanation: The patient's stage 3 pressure ulcer on the sacral region should be dressed with hydrocolloid hydrogel with foam dressing gauze.
This type of dressing provides a moist wound environment, which is essential for optimal healing. A moist environment supports cell migration, reduces pain, and minimizes scab formation, facilitating faster healing. Hydrocolloid and foam dressings are designed to absorb excess wound exudate, which is common in stage 3 pressure ulcers. By managing the exudate, the dressing helps prevent maceration and keeps the wound bed clean.
Foam dressings offer protection and cushioning, reducing pressure on the ulcerated area. This is particularly important for sacral pressure ulcers, which are prone to pressure and friction.
The hydrogel component helps to maintain moisture and soothe the wound, thereby reducing pain during dressing changes.

Que 3. What is the purpose of repositioning immobile patients every 2 hours?

A. To prevent pressure ulcers
B. To help the patient sleep better
C. To monitor the patient's breathing
D. To check the patient's vitals

Answer 3:
 A. To prevent pressure ulcers

Explanation: Repositioning immobile patients every 2 hours helps to prevent pressure ulcers by reducing the pressure on one area of the skin for an extended period of time. This helps to maintain normal skin integrity and reduces the risk of developing pressure ulcers.

Que 4. What is the definition of Pressure Ulcer?

A) Any damage to normal skin due to underlying bones
 B) Any damage to skin due to external surface friction
C) Any damage to skin due to pressure from external surface
D) Any damage to normal skin due to internal pressure

A pressure ulcer (also known as a bedsore) is localized damage to the skin and underlying tissue, usually over a bony prominence, caused by prolonged pressure or a combination of pressure, shear, and friction. These ulcers commonly occur in individuals with limited mobility, such as bedridden or wheelchair-bound patients.

Que 5. What is the first stage of Pressure Ulcer?

 A) Red intact skin with no wounds
B) Some abrasion and visibility of subcutaneous skin
C) Dermis part is lost and forms sunken hole
D) Full skin is lost opening underlying muscles, tendons or bones

Answer 5: A) Red intact skin with no wounds

Explanation: The first stage of pressure ulcer is defined as red intact skin with no wounds. The skin may be warm or cool, firm or soft and does not turn white when pressed. This is a sign that a pressure ulcer may be forming.

Que 6. What is the appropriate dressing for each stage of pressure ulcer?

A) For stage 1: Hydrocolloid Hydrogel with foam dressing Gauze
B) For stage 2: Nontransparent hydrocolloid dressing
C) For stage 3: Composite film hydrocolloid dressing and hydrogels
D) For stage 4: Calcium alginate gauze
E) For unstageable: Hydrocolloid Hydrogel with foam dressing Gauze
F) For deep tissue injury: Nontransport hydrocolloid dressing
G) For stage 1: Composite film hydrocolloid dressing and hydrogels
H) For deep tissue injury: Surgical interventions and adherent film gauze

Ans 6: B and H

Explanation: B) For stage 2: Nontransport hydrocolloid dressing is correct. This type of dressing is painless in removal and is waterproof. The affected area should be cleaned every day. H) For deep tissue injury: Surgical interventions and adherent film gauze is correct. Surgical interventions may be needed along with adherent film gauze for unstageable and sometimes for deep tissue injury.

CASE STUDY 11: Management Approaches for Rheumatoid Arthritis

Patient's History: A 56-year-old male presents with joint pain and swelling in both hands and feet for the past 6 months. He reports morning stiffness lasting for 1 hour and difficulty in performing daily activities. He has a history of smoking for 20 years and reports no other significant medical history.

Nurse's Notes:
- Joints in both hands and feet are swollen and tender to touch
- Morning stiffness lasting for 1 hour
- Difficulty in performing daily activities
- Positive history of smoking for 20 years

Medications:

Ibuprofen
Dosage: Typically, 400 mg to 800 mg every 6 to 8 hours as needed.
Methotrexate
Dosage: Typically, once a week, starting with a low dose and titrating as needed.

Lab Values:
- Rheumatoid Factor: Positive
- ESR: Elevated
- X-rays: Show signs of joint destruction and ankyloses

Que 1. What is the most likely diagnosis for the patient based on the information provided?

A. Osteoarthritis
B. Rheumatoid Arthritis
C. Gout
D. Lupus

Ans 1:

Explanation: A. Osteoarthritis is a degenerative joint disease that is usually seen in older individuals and is not associated with elevated ESR or positive rheumatoid factor.
B. Rheumatoid Arthritis is the most likely diagnosis as it presents with symmetrical joint swelling, morning stiffness, difficulty in performing daily activities, elevated ESR, and positive rheumatoid factor.
C. Gout is a type of arthritis caused by the buildup of uric acid crystals in the joints and is not associated with elevated ESR or positive rheumatoid factor.
D. Lupus is an autoimmune disease that can present with joint pain and swelling but is not typically associated with a positive rheumatoid factor or elevated ESR.

Que 2. The primary goal of nursing management for patients with rheumatoid arthritis (RA) is to _____.
a) promote rest and immobilization of affected joints
b) provide passive range of motion exercises to affected joints
c) administer corticosteroids to reduce inflammation and pain
d) facilitate patient self-management and maximize functional ability

Ans 2:

Correct answer: d) facilitate patient self-management and maximize functional ability

Explanation: RA is a chronic autoimmune disease characterized by joint inflammation and destruction, leading to pain, stiffness, and functional impairment. The primary goal of nursing management for patients with RA is to facilitate patient self-management and maximize functional ability. This includes educating patients on the disease process, medications, and self-care strategies, such as exercise and joint protection techniques, to help them manage their symptoms and maintain their independence.

Option a) promote rest and immobilization of affected joints is not the best approach as prolonged immobilization can lead to muscle weakness, joint stiffness, and contractures. Rest is essential during acute flare-ups, but too much rest can lead to muscle atrophy, which can exacerbate symptoms.

Option b) provide passive range of motion exercises to affected joints is not an appropriate nursing intervention for RA as it can exacerbate inflammation and pain. Active range of motion exercises are preferred as they can improve joint mobility and muscle strength without aggravating symptoms.

Option c) administer corticosteroids to reduce inflammation and pain is a medical intervention and is not the primary goal of nursing management for RA. However, nurses can monitor patients for adverse effects of corticosteroids, such as hyperglycemia, hypertension, and gastrointestinal distress.

Option d) facilitate patient self-management and maximize functional ability is the correct answer as it aligns with the current trend in managing RA, which is patient-centered care. RA can affect many aspects of a patient's life, and nursing interventions should focus on addressing these issues to help patients manage their symptoms and maintain their quality of life.

Que 3. Why was the patient ordered to have an Erythrocyte Sedimentation Rate (ESR) test?

A. To evaluate for anemia
B. To monitor the patient's response to treatment
C. To evaluate for inflammation
D. To evaluate for joint destruction

Ans 3:

Explanation: C. The ESR test is ordered to evaluate for inflammation as it is a non-specific test that measures the rate at which red blood cells settle in a test tube and is elevated in conditions that cause inflammation, such as Rheumatoid Arthritis. A. Anemia is not indicated based on the patient's history and symptoms.
B. The ESR test is not specifically used to monitor the patient's response to treatment.
D. The X-rays were ordered to evaluate for joint destruction, not the ESR test.

Que 4. What is the purpose of prescribing NSAIDs for the patient?

A. To relieve joint pain
B. To reduce inflammation
C. To slow down the progression of joint destruction
D. To treat the underlying cause of the disease

Ans 4:

Explanation: A. The NSAIDs (ibuprofen) are prescribed to relieve joint pain and reduce inflammation, which is a common symptom of Rheumatoid Arthritis.
B. NSAIDs are commonly used to reduce inflammation in conditions such as Rheumatoid Arthritis.
C. NSAIDs do not slow down the progression of joint destruction, they only relieve pain and reduce inflammation.
D. NSAIDs do not treat the underlying cause of the disease, they only relieve symptoms.

Que 5. Which instruction should the nurse prioritize when teaching a patient with rheumatoid arthritis (RA)?

Options: A) Engage in high-impact aerobic exercise to improve overall fitness
B) Take over-the-counter (OTC) nonsteroidal anti-inflammatory drugs (NSAIDs) daily
C) Follow a balanced diet that includes omega-3 fatty acids and antioxidants
D) Report any new or worsening joint pain to the healthcare provider immediately

Ans 5:

Correct Answer: D) Report any new or worsening joint pain to the healthcare provider immediately

Explanation: A) Engage in high-impact aerobic exercise to improve overall fitness: This option is incorrect. While exercise is beneficial for patients with RA, high-impact exercises can put too much pressure on joints and cause further damage. Low-impact exercises like walking, swimming, or cycling are better suited for patients with RA.

B) Take over-the-counter (OTC) nonsteroidal anti-inflammatory drugs (NSAIDs) daily: This option is incorrect. Although OTC NSAIDs can help to alleviate pain and inflammation in patients with RA, it's important to follow the healthcare provider's instructions regarding their use, as they can cause gastrointestinal side effects and other complications with prolonged use.

C) Follow a balanced diet that includes omega-3 fatty acids and antioxidants: This option is partially correct. A balanced diet that includes omega-3 fatty acids and antioxidants can help to reduce inflammation and improve overall health in patients with RA. However, it's not the priority instruction for a patient with RA.

D) Report any new or worsening joint pain to the healthcare provider immediately: This option is correct. Patients with RA are at risk for joint damage and deformities if their condition is not managed properly. Therefore, it's crucial for patients to report any new or worsening joint pain to their healthcare provider immediately, so that prompt treatment can be initiated.

Que 6. In rheumatoid arthritis, which of the following joints are typically affected, and what is the most effective way for a nurse to instruct the patient in managing pain associated with these joints?

A) Only weight-bearing joints such as knees and hips are affected, and the patient should apply heat to these areas to manage pain.
B) Both weight-bearing and non-weight-bearing joints such as hands and wrists are affected, and the patient should apply cold compresses to these areas to manage pain.
C) Only non-weight-bearing joints such as hands and wrists are affected, and the patient should perform gentle stretching exercises to manage pain.
D) Both weight-bearing and non-weight-bearing joints such as knees, hips, hands, and wrists are affected, and the patient should use a combination of both heat and cold therapies to manage pain.

Ans 6:

D) Both weight-bearing and non-weight-bearing joints such as knees, hips, hands, and wrists are affected, and the patient should use a combination of both heat and cold therapies to manage pain.

Explanation: Rheumatoid arthritis can affect both weight-bearing and non-weight-bearing joints in the body, including the hands, wrists, knees, and hips. Therefore, option A and C are incorrect. The most effective way for a nurse to instruct the patient in managing pain associated with these joints is to use a combination of both heat and cold therapies, as both can provide relief to different types of pain. Heat can help relax stiff muscles and increase blood flow to the affected areas, while cold therapy can reduce inflammation and swelling. Therefore, option B is incorrect, and the correct answer is D. In addition to using heat and cold therapies, the patient may also benefit from taking pain medications as prescribed by their healthcare provider and performing gentle exercises to maintain joint mobility.

CASE STUDY 12: Diagnosis and Management of Adrenal Insufficiency

Patient Case Study: A 38-year-old female presents with symptoms of salt cravings, irregular menstrual cycle, fatigue, and weakness. The patient also reports experiencing weight loss and postural hypotension.

Nurse's Notes:
Assessed patient's vital signs (BP: 100/60 mmHg, HR: 90 bpm, RR: 18 breaths/min)
Patient reported salt cravings, irregular menstrual cycle, fatigue, and weakness
Observed skin pigmentation and reported weight loss and postural hypotension
Reviewed patient's lab results, including high Calcium and Potassium levels, and low sodium levels

Medications
Fludrocortisone:
 Dosage: Typically, 0.05-0.2 mg once daily.

Lab Values:
Sodium (Na): 130 mEq/L (normal range: 135-145 mEq/L)
Potassium (K): 5.0 mEq/L (normal range: 3.5-5.0 mEq/L)
Calcium (Ca): 10.2 mg/dL (normal range: 8.5-10.5 mg/dL)

Que 1. What is the most likely diagnosis for the patient in this case study based on the presented symptoms and lab results?

A. Hypothyroidism
B. Addison's disease
C. Hyperparathyroidism
D. Cushing's syndrome

Ans 1:

Answer: B. Addison's disease

Explanation:
Option A: Hypothyroidism can cause fatigue, weight gain, and dry skin, but it does not typically cause salt cravings or high calcium levels.
Option B: Addison's disease, a condition where the adrenal gland does not produce enough hormones, presents with symptoms such as salt cravings, irregular menstrual cycle, fatigue, weakness, weight loss, and postural hypotension.
Option C: Hyperparathyroidism is a condition in which the parathyroid glands produce too much parathyroid hormone, causing high calcium levels. It does not typically cause salt cravings or postural hypotension.
Option D: Cushing's syndrome is a condition in which the body produces too much cortisol. It can cause weight gain, fatigue, and weakness, but it does not typically present with salt cravings, postural hypotension, or low sodium levels.

Que 2. The nurse notes that the patient has salt carvings. **Why may a patient with Addison's disease crave salt?**

A) Low levels of cortisol increase sodium excretion, leading to salt cravings.
B) High levels of aldosterone increase sodium excretion, leading to salt cravings.
C) Low levels of aldosterone decrease sodium excretion, leading to salt cravings.
D) High levels of cortisol decrease sodium excretion, leading to salt cravings.

Ans 2:

Answer: C) Low levels of aldosterone decrease sodium excretion, leading to salt cravings.

Explanation: Addison's disease is a condition in which the adrenal glands do not produce enough cortisol and aldosterone. Aldosterone is a hormone produced by the adrenal glands that regulates the body's sodium and potassium balance. It does this by increasing the reabsorption of sodium by the kidneys, leading to increased blood volume and blood pressure. In Addison's disease, the lack of aldosterone leads to decreased sodium reabsorption and increased sodium excretion by the kidneys, which can cause a decrease in blood volume and blood pressure.

Salt craving is a common symptom in patients with Addison's disease because the body is trying to compensate for the low levels of aldosterone by increasing salt intake. The body needs more salt to maintain its sodium balance, and this craving is a result of the body's attempt to maintain homeostasis.

Option A is incorrect because low levels of cortisol do not increase sodium excretion; rather, they decrease it by decreasing the glomerular filtration rate (GFR) in the kidneys, leading to decreased urine output and increased sodium reabsorption. Option B is incorrect because high levels of aldosterone increase sodium reabsorption, not sodium excretion, which would lead to decreased sodium levels in the blood, and thus not cause salt cravings. Option D is also incorrect because high levels of cortisol do not decrease sodium excretion; rather, they increase it by increasing the GFR in the kidneys, leading to increased urine output and decreased sodium reabsorption. Therefore, the correct answer is option C.

Que 3. Which of the following lab values is commonly seen in individuals with Addison's disease?

A) Elevated serum sodium
B) Elevated serum potassium
C) Elevated serum cortisol
D) Elevated serum aldosterone

Ans 3:

The correct answer is B) Elevated serum potassium.

In Addison's disease, the adrenal glands do not produce enough cortisol and aldosterone, leading to low levels of these hormones and an increase in potassium levels.

Que 3. Which of the following properties are associated with Addison's disease?

A) Hypercortisolism
B) Hypotension
C) Hyperpigmentation
D) Moon facies
E) Hirsutism
F) Hypokalemia
G) Hypernatremia
H) Weight gain

Ans 4:
The properties associated with Addison's disease are:
B) Hypotension C) Hyperpigmentation
Explanation:
- **Hypotension:** Addison's disease is characterized by insufficient production of adrenal hormones (cortisol and aldosterone), which can lead to low blood pressure (hypotension).
- **Hyperpigmentation:** One of the hallmark signs of Addison's disease is hyperpigmentation, especially in areas exposed to friction, such as the knuckles, elbows, and knees. This occurs due to increased production of adrenocorticotropic hormone (ACTH), which stimulates melanin production.

Other Options:
- **A) Hypercortisolism:** This is associated with Cushing's syndrome, not Addison's disease.
- **D) Moon facies:** This is a characteristic feature of Cushing's syndrome, not Addison's disease.
- **E) Hirsutism:** This is associated with conditions that involve excessive androgen production, such as polycystic ovary syndrome (PCOS) or Cushing's syndrome.
- **F) Hypokalemia:** Addison's disease typically presents with hyperkalemia (elevated potassium levels) due to aldosterone deficiency, not hypokalemia.

- **G) Hypernatremia:** Addison's disease usually involves hyponatremia (low sodium levels) due to aldosterone deficiency, not hypernatremia.
- **H) Weight gain:** Addison's disease is more commonly associated with weight loss, not weight gain.

Que 5. Which of the following is the most appropriate nursing intervention for a patient with Addison's disease experiencing an acute adrenal crisis?

A) Administering IV fluids containing dextrose
B) Administering high doses of glucocorticoids
C) Administering a potassium-sparing diuretic
D) Administering beta-adrenergic blockers

Ans 5:

Explanation:

An acute adrenal crisis can occur when the patient experiences a sudden and severe worsening of symptoms due to stress or illness. Nursing management of a patient with Addison's disease during an acute adrenal crisis is critical, and it involves prompt intervention to prevent life-threatening complications.

A) Administering IV fluids containing dextrose: This option is partially correct as it addresses the fluid and electrolyte imbalances that can occur during an acute adrenal crisis. Addison's disease patients may experience hypotension, dehydration, and hyponatremia, which can be corrected with the administration of fluids containing dextrose. However, this option does not address the underlying cause of the crisis.

B) Administering high doses of glucocorticoids: This option is the correct answer as it addresses the underlying cause of the crisis, which is the lack of cortisol production. Patients with Addison's disease need lifelong replacement therapy with glucocorticoids, and during an acute adrenal crisis, high doses of glucocorticoids are necessary to prevent life-threatening complications such as hypotension, shock, and renal failure.

C) Administering a potassium-sparing diuretic: This option is incorrect as it does not address the underlying cause of the crisis. Potassium-sparing diuretics are used to treat hypertension and edema and can be harmful to patients with Addison's disease who are already experiencing electrolyte imbalances.

D) Administering beta-adrenergic blockers: This option is incorrect as it can worsen the patient's condition. Beta-adrenergic blockers are contraindicated in patients with Addison's disease as they can mask the signs and symptoms of hypoglycemia, which can be life-threatening in these patients. Furthermore, beta-adrenergic blockers can exacerbate the hypotension that occurs during an acute adrenal crisis.

Que 6. Which of the following conditions can cause high potassium levels in the blood?

A) Hyperparathyroidism
B) Addison's disease
C) Chronic kidney disease
D) Diabetic ketoacidosis

Ans 6: B, C, D

Conditions B, C, and D can cause high potassium levels in the blood (hyperkalemia):

- B) Addison's disease: Low aldosterone levels lead to reduced potassium excretion by the kidneys, resulting in hyperkalemia.
- C) Chronic kidney disease: Impaired renal function reduces the kidneys' ability to excrete potassium, leading to hyperkalemia.
- D) Diabetic ketoacidosis: Insulin deficiency and acidosis cause potassium to shift out of cells into the bloodstream, resulting in hyperkalemia.

    A) Hyperparathyroidism primarily affects calcium levels and does not typically cause high potassium levels.

CASE STUDY 13: Hypothyroidism Diagnosis and Management

Jane is a 45-year-old female who presents with a chief complaint of fatigue and weight gain over the past few months. She reports feeling cold all the time and has noticed that her skin has become dry and her hair has become brittle. She denies any significant medical history and is currently not taking any medications.

Nurse's Notes: Upon assessment, Jane appears pale and fatigued. Her vital signs are within normal limits, except for a slightly elevated blood pressure of 138/84 mmHg. She reports a 10-pound weight gain over the past 6 months, despite maintaining a healthy diet and exercise routine. Her skin is dry, and her hair is thin and brittle. She also reports feeling cold all the time. Physical examination of the thyroid gland reveals a diffuse enlargement of the gland with no nodules or tenderness.

Medications

Levothyroxine (Synthroid, Levoxyl):

Dosage: The typical starting dose is 25-50 mcg once daily

Liothyronine (Cytomel):

Dosage: The usual starting dose is 5-25 mcg once or twice daily.

Lab Values: TSH: 5.5 uIU/mL (normal range 0.5-5.0 uIU/mL)
Free T4: 0.8 ng/dL (normal range 0.8-1.8 ng/dL)
Free T3: 2.5 pg/mL (normal range 2.3-4.2 pg/mL)

Que 1. What is the most likely diagnosis for Jane based on her presentation and lab values?
A) Hyperthyroidism
B) Hypothyroidism
C) Subclinical hyperthyroidism
D) Normal thyroid function

Answer 1:

B) Hypothyroidism

Explanation:

Jane's presentation of fatigue, weight gain, cold intolerance, dry skin, and brittle hair, along with a diffuse enlargement of the thyroid gland, are all consistent with a diagnosis of hypothyroidism. Her TSH level is elevated at 5.5 uIU/mL, which indicates decreased thyroid hormone production and is a hallmark finding in hypothyroidism. Additionally, her free T4 level is at the lower end of the normal range, while her free T3 level is slightly decreased, further supporting a diagnosis of hypothyroidism.

Option A) Hyperthyroidism is incorrect because Jane's presentation is not consistent with an overactive thyroid gland. Hyperthyroidism typically presents with symptoms such as weight loss, heat intolerance, palpitations, and tremors, and lab values show a decreased TSH level and increased levels of free T4 and/or free T3.

Option C) Subclinical hyperthyroidism is also incorrect because Jane's TSH level is elevated, indicating decreased thyroid hormone production, rather than decreased TSH production. Subclinical hyperthyroidism is characterized by a slightly decreased TSH level with normal levels of free T4 and free T3.
Option D) Normal thyroid function is incorrect because Jane's TSH level is outside the normal range, indicating abnormal thyroid function. Normal thyroid function is characterized by TSH, free T4, and free T3 levels within the normal range.

Therefore, based on Jane's presentation and lab values, the most likely diagnosis is hypothyroidism.

Que 2. Which of the following is characterized by weight gain, fatigue, and a diffuse enlargement of the thyroid gland?
A) Hypothyroidism
B) Hyperthyroidism
C) Thyroid storm
D) Both A and C

Answer 2:
Hypothyroidism

Explanation:

Hypothyroidism is a condition where the thyroid gland does not produce enough thyroid hormones, resulting in a slowing down of the body's metabolic processes. This is characterized by symptoms such as weight gain, fatigue, constipation, cold intolerance, and dry skin. Additionally, a physical examination may reveal a diffuse enlargement of the thyroid gland, also known as a goiter, which can occur due to increased stimulation of the thyroid gland in an attempt to produce more hormones. Therefore, option A) Hypothyroidism is the correct answer.

Option B) Hyperthyroidism is characterized by an overactive thyroid gland, resulting in the body's metabolic processes speeding up. Symptoms may include weight loss, anxiety, tremors, heat intolerance, and palpitations. Physical examination may reveal an enlarged thyroid gland, but it is typically accompanied by nodules and tenderness, rather than a diffuse enlargement.

Option C) Thyroid storm is a severe complication of hyperthyroidism characterized by fever, tachycardia, hypertension, altered mental status, and possible organ failure. This is a medical emergency and requires immediate treatment in an intensive care setting. It is not characterized by weight gain or a diffuse enlargement of the thyroid gland.

Option D) Both A and C is incorrect because although hypothyroidism and thyroid storm are both related to thyroid dysfunction, they are opposite ends of the spectrum in terms of severity and presentation. Thyroid storm is a medical emergency characterized by extreme hyperthyroidism, while hypothyroidism is a chronic condition characterized by decreased thyroid hormone production.

Therefore, based on the symptoms provided, the correct answer is A) Hypothyroidism.

Que 3. If the patient's conditions worsen, what is the priority nursing intervention for a patient experiencing myxedema coma due to hypothyroidism?

A) Administer thyroid replacement hormone therapy
B) Administer vasopressor medications to treat hypotension
C) Administer corticosteroids to reduce inflammation
D) Administer oxygen therapy to treat respiratory distress

Ans 3:
Correct answer: A) Administer thyroid replacement hormone therapy

Explanation: Myxedema coma is a rare, life-threatening complication of hypothyroidism characterized by severe hypothyroidism leading to decreased metabolism and altered mental status. The priority nursing intervention for a patient experiencing myxedema coma is to administer thyroid replacement hormone therapy to correct the hypothyroidism and prevent further complications. Administering vasopressor medications to treat hypotension, corticosteroids to reduce inflammation, or oxygen therapy to treat respiratory distress may be appropriate interventions but are not the priority in this situation. The primary goal is to treat the underlying hypothyroidism to prevent further complications and improve the patient's overall condition.

Que 4. Which of the following is the most appropriate nursing intervention for a patient experiencing thyrotoxicosis crisis?

A) Administer a high dose of levothyroxine to rapidly decrease thyroid hormone levels.
B) Place the patient in a cool environment to decrease metabolic demands.
C) Administer a beta-blocker to decrease heart rate and blood pressure.
D) Encourage the patient to consume a high-protein diet to promote healing.

Ans 4:

Correct answer: C) Administer a beta-blocker to decrease heart rate and blood pressure.

Explanation: Thyrotoxicosis crisis, also known as thyroid storm, is a life-threatening complication of hyperthyroidism. Symptoms include fever, tachycardia, hypertension, and altered mental status. Treatment involves managing the symptoms while decreasing thyroid hormone levels. Administering a beta-blocker, such as propranolol, is the most appropriate nursing intervention because it will decrease heart rate and blood pressure, reducing the risk of cardiovascular complications. Option A is incorrect because levothyroxine would further increase thyroid hormone levels and exacerbate the crisis. Option B is incorrect because although a cool environment may help reduce symptoms, it does not address the underlying cause of the crisis. Option D is incorrect because a high-protein diet would not directly address the symptoms of thyrotoxicosis crisis.

Que 5. Which of the following is an appropriate nursing intervention for managing constipation, a common complication of hypothyroidism, with diet?

A. Increasing intake of high-fiber foods
B. Decreasing fluid intake to avoid further fluid retention
C. Avoiding foods rich in iron and calcium
D. Increasing intake of caffeine-containing beverages

Ans 5:
Correct answer: A. Increasing intake of high-fiber foods

Explanation: Constipation is a common complication of hypothyroidism due to the decreased metabolic rate in the body. One of the nursing interventions to manage constipation in hypothyroidism is to increase the intake of high-fiber foods such as fruits, vegetables, and whole grains. This will help to promote bowel movement and prevent constipation. Option B is incorrect because decreasing fluid intake may lead to dehydration and worsen constipation. Option C is incorrect because iron and calcium-rich foods are important for patients with hypothyroidism. Option D is incorrect because caffeine-containing beverages may cause dehydration and interfere with the absorption of thyroid medications.

Que 6: Which of the following are good choices for education that should be given by a nurse to a patient who is suffering from hypothyroidism? Select all that apply.

A. Importance of taking thyroid hormone replacement medication as prescribed
B. Maintaining a healthy and balanced diet
C. Avoiding over-the-counter supplements without consulting a healthcare provider
D. Importance of regular exercise to manage weight
E. Monitoring thyroid hormone levels regularly
F. Avoiding exposure to extreme temperatures
G. Using iodized salt for cooking

Ans 6:

Correct answers: A, B, C, D, E, F.

Explanation:
A. Importance of taking thyroid hormone replacement medication as prescribed
- Adherence to medication is crucial for managing thyroid hormone levels and symptoms.

B. Maintaining a healthy and balanced diet
- Proper nutrition supports overall health and can help manage symptoms.

C. Avoiding over-the-counter supplements without consulting a healthcare provider
- Some supplements may interfere with thyroid hormone levels or medications.

D. Importance of regular exercise to manage weight
- Regular exercise helps maintain a healthy weight and supports overall well-being.

E. Monitoring thyroid hormone levels regularly
- Regular monitoring ensures that medication dosage is appropriate and effective.

F. Avoiding exposure to extreme temperatures
- Patients with hypothyroidism may be more sensitive to cold and heat, so avoiding extreme temperatures is important for comfort and health.

CASE STUDY 14 : Diagnosis and Management of Type 2 Diabetes Mellitus

Patient Information:

Name: Mr. Pavlo Smith
Age: 55 years
Gender: Male
Occupation: Office Manager
Medical History: Hypertension, Hyperlipidemia

Presenting Complaint:

Mr. Smith presents to the clinic with complaints of increased thirst, frequent urination, and unexplained weight loss over the past few weeks. He reports feeling fatigued and has noticed blurred vision on several occasions.

Nurse's Notes:

History:

Mr. Smith has a medical history significant for hypertension and hyperlipidemia.
No history of major surgeries.
Social history: Non-smoker, occasional alcohol use, sedentary lifestyle.

Physical Examination:

General Appearance: Appears tired, slightly overweight.
Eyes: Fundoscopic exam reveals early signs of diabetic retinopathy.
Skin: Dry skin, no evidence of wounds or infections.
Neurological: No focal deficits, but diminished vibratory sensation in lower extremities.

Vital Signs:

Blood Pressure: 140/90 mmHg
Heart Rate: 82 bpm
Respiratory Rate: 18 breaths/min
Temperature: 98.6°F (37°C)
Oxygen Saturation: 98% on room air

Laboratory Results:

Fasting Blood Glucose: 210 mg/dL (Normal: 70-100 mg/dL)
Hemoglobin A1c: 9.5% (Normal: <5.7%)
Lipid Profile: Elevated LDL cholesterol (160 mg/dL), elevated triglycerides (200 mg/dL), decreased HDL cholesterol (35 mg/dL).
Creatinine: 1.0 mg/dL (Normal: 0.5-1.2 mg/dL)
Urine Analysis: Positive for glucosuria and ketonuria.

Que 1:

Based on the provided information, what is the right condition that Mr. Pavlo Smith is likely suffering from?

Hypertension
Hyperlipidemia
Diabetic Retinopathy
Type 2 Diabetes Mellitus
Chronic Kidney Disease

Ans 1:
Explanation:

Correct Answer: 4. Type 2 Diabetes Mellitus

Why it's the right answer:

Mr. Pavlo Smith is likely suffering from Type 2 Diabetes Mellitus based on the following findings:

Increased thirst, frequent urination, and unexplained weight loss are classic symptoms of diabetes.
Fatigue and blurred vision are also common symptoms associated with uncontrolled diabetes.
Elevated fasting blood glucose of 210 mg/dL and a high Hemoglobin A1c of 9.5% indicate poor glycemic control, characteristic of diabetes.
Positive findings in urine analysis for glucosuria and ketonuria further support the diagnosis of diabetes. The fundoscopic exam revealing early signs of diabetic retinopathy is a complication associated with diabetes.

Hypertension: Mr. Smith has a history of hypertension, but the symptoms (increased thirst, frequent urination, unexplained weight loss) and the abnormal laboratory findings (elevated blood glucose, high Hemoglobin A1c) are more indicative of diabetes.

Hyperlipidemia: While Mr. Smith has hyperlipidemia, the constellation of symptoms and laboratory findings is more suggestive of diabetes.

Diabetic Retinopathy: Diabetic retinopathy is mentioned in the nurse's notes, but it is a complication of diabetes rather than the primary condition causing the symptoms.

Chronic Kidney Disease: While the creatinine level is mentioned and is within the normal range, the symptoms and laboratory findings are more indicative of uncontrolled diabetes rather than chronic kidney disease at this point. However, chronic kidney disease can be a complication of long-term uncontrolled diabetes.

Que 2:
Fill in the blanks with correct option.
Patients prescribed _____ should be advised to monitor for symptoms of heart failure, such as shortness of breath and swelling in the legs.
A. Metformin B. Insulin C. Thiazolidinediones D. Sulfonylureas

Patients prescribed **C. Thiazolidinediones** should be advised to monitor for symptoms of heart failure, such as shortness of breath and swelling in the legs.

Explanation: Thiazolidinediones (such as pioglitazone and rosiglitazone) are associated with an increased risk of heart failure. Therefore, patients taking these medications should be aware of and monitor for symptoms of heart failure.

Note: The next 4 questions are nearly the same. The idea is to show how same question could be asked in different ways and formats.

Ans 3:

Which of the following statements from a nurse is NOT appropriate in the nursing management of a patient with Type 2 Diabetes Mellitus?

Options:

"You should aim to maintain a healthy weight through a balanced diet and regular exercise."
"It's important to monitor your blood glucose levels regularly to ensure they stay within the target range."
"Skipping meals occasionally can help control blood sugar levels."
"Take your prescribed medications as directed, even if you feel well."
"If you experience symptoms of hypoglycemia, consume a sugary snack or drink to raise your blood sugar."
"Smoking cessation is crucial for managing diabetes and reducing cardiovascular risk."
"Limit your fluid intake to avoid excessive thirst and urination."
Explanation:

Ans 3:

Correct Answer: 3. "Skipping meals occasionally can help control blood sugar levels."

Encouraging the patient to skip meals is not appropriate in the management of Type 2 Diabetes Mellitus. Consistent, balanced meals are crucial for managing blood glucose levels. Skipping meals can lead to hypoglycemia or overeating later, causing blood sugar fluctuations.

Other options:

"You should aim to maintain a healthy weight through a balanced diet and regular exercise." - Correct: Promoting a healthy weight through diet and exercise is essential for diabetes management.

"It's important to monitor your blood glucose levels regularly to ensure they stay within the target range." - Correct: Regular monitoring helps in maintaining glycemic control and adjusting treatment as needed.

"Take your prescribed medications as directed, even if you feel well." - Correct: Medication adherence is crucial for managing blood glucose levels and preventing complications.

"If you experience symptoms of hypoglycemia, consume a sugary snack or drink to raise your blood sugar." - Correct: This advice is appropriate for managing hypoglycemic episodes.

"Smoking cessation is crucial for managing diabetes and reducing cardiovascular risk." - Correct: Smoking cessation is important for overall cardiovascular health and complements diabetes management.

"Limit your fluid intake to avoid excessive thirst and urination." - Correct: While monitoring fluid intake is important, advising strict limitation may not be appropriate. Adequate hydration is generally encouraged unless otherwise contraindicated.

Que 4:

The following is a nurse's advice on the case. Highlight the advices which are not correct:

Managing diabetes requires careful adherence to medical advice. Doctors recommend maintaining a healthy weight through a balanced diet and regular exercise. Regular monitoring of blood glucose levels is essential to ensure they stay within the target range. Skipping meals occasionally is advised to help control blood sugar levels and prevent overeating. Taking prescribed medications as directed, even if the patient feels well, is crucial for managing blood glucose levels and preventing complications. In case of hypoglycemia symptoms, patients should consume a sugary snack or drink to raise blood sugar. Smoking cessation is highly recommended to manage diabetes and reduce cardiovascular risk. Limiting fluid intake is suggested to avoid excessive thirst and urination.

Ans 4:
Right Answers:

The doctor recommends maintaining a healthy weight through a balanced diet and regular exercise.
Regular monitoring of blood glucose levels is essential to ensure they stay within the target range.
Taking prescribed medications as directed, even if the patient feels well, is crucial for managing blood glucose levels and preventing complications.
In case of hypoglycemia symptoms, patients should consume a sugary snack or drink to raise blood sugar.
Smoking cessation is highly recommended to manage diabetes and reduce cardiovascular risk.

Wrong Answers and Explanations:

"Skipping meals occasionally is advised to help control blood sugar levels and prevent overeating." (Wrong): Skipping meals is not advised; consistent, balanced meals are crucial for managing blood glucose levels.
"Limiting fluid intake is suggested to avoid excessive thirst and urination." (Wrong): Adequate hydration is generally encouraged unless otherwise contraindicated; limiting fluids may lead to dehydration and other health issues.
The wrong options aim to mislead, emphasizing the importance of accurate information for effective diabetes management.

Que 5:

Select if the row contains 'correct' or 'incorrect' information:

Management of Diabetes	Explanation
Maintain a healthy weight through diet and exercise.	Regular physical activity and a balanced diet are crucial for managing weight and improving insulin sensitivity in diabetes.
Monitor blood glucose levels regularly.	Regular monitoring helps in understanding and managing blood glucose levels, enabling timely adjustments to treatment plans.

Skipping meals occasionally aids in blood sugar control.	Sometimes when the blood sugar shoots up, skipping meal could be a good choice to keep the level of blood sugar normal.
Take prescribed medications as directed, even if feeling well.	Medication adherence is essential for maintaining stable blood glucose levels and preventing complications associated with diabetes.
Consume a sugary snack to raise blood sugar in case of hypoglycemia.	In the event of low blood sugar, consuming a sugary snack or drink helps raise blood sugar levels and manage hypoglycemic symptoms effectively.
Smoking cessation is crucial for managing diabetes and reducing cardiovascular risk.	Quitting smoking is essential for overall cardiovascular health and complements diabetes management by reducing associated risks.
Limit fluid intake to avoid excessive thirst and urination.	While monitoring fluid intake is important, this statement is incorrect. Adequate hydration is generally encouraged unless otherwise contraindicated in diabetes management.

Que :

Which row contains incorrect information in the management of diabetes?

Ans 5:

Explanation:

The row with "Skipping meals occasionally aids in blood sugar control" contains incorrect information. Skipping meals can lead to blood sugar fluctuations, potentially causing hypoglycemia or overeating later. Consistent, balanced meals are crucial for glycemic control in diabetes. All other rows provide accurate guidance for managing diabetes, emphasizing the importance of a healthy lifestyle, regular monitoring, medication adherence, and appropriate responses to hypoglycemic episodes.

Que 6:

Which of the following statements by the patient indicates the need for counseling regarding diabetes management?

Options:

"I check my blood glucose levels regularly and record the results in a logbook."
"I occasionally forget to take my prescribed diabetes medications."
"I engage in moderate-intensity exercise for at least 30 minutes most days of the week."
"I follow a well-balanced diet with a mix of carbohydrates, proteins, and healthy fats."
"I usually consume sugary snacks between meals to keep my energy up."
"I quit smoking as soon as I was diagnosed with diabetes."
"I limit my alcohol intake to one drink per day as recommended by my healthcare provider."
"I understand the importance of maintaining a healthy weight for managing diabetes."
"I skip meals occasionally to control my blood sugar levels."
"I have an emergency kit with glucose tablets in case my blood sugar drops unexpectedly."

Ans 6:

Explanation:

Correct Answers:

Option 2: Forgetting to take prescribed diabetes medications can have a significant impact on glycemic control and warrants counseling.

Option 5: Consuming sugary snacks between meals may contribute to blood sugar fluctuations and requires counseling for better dietary choices.

Option 9: Skipping meals to control blood sugar levels is not recommended and necessitates counseling on the importance of regular, balanced meals.

Incorrect Answers:

Options 1, 3, 4, 6, 7, 8, and 10: These statements indicate positive behaviors such as regular monitoring, engaging in exercise, following a balanced diet, quitting smoking, limiting alcohol intake, understanding the importance of maintaining a healthy weight, and being prepared with an emergency kit, respectively. While further education may be beneficial, they do not specifically indicate a need for counseling on diabetes management.

CASE STUDY 15: Anxiety Disorders and Cardiovascular Health

Patient History:
Mr. Vimal, a 32-year-old male, presents to the emergency department (ED) with complaints of chest pain, shortness of breath, and dizziness. He reports a history of generalized anxiety disorder (GAD) and mentions that he has been under increased stress due to work-related issues.

Nurse Notes:
Upon assessment, Mr. Vimal appears restless, fidgety, and reports difficulty concentrating. He frequently checks his pulse and expresses fear of having a heart attack. He denies any recent trauma or substance use. The nurse observes increased muscle tension, rapid speech, and trembling hands.

Medication List and Doses:

Alprazolam (Xanax): 0.5 mg orally every 8 hours as needed for anxiety.
Escitalopram (Lexapro): 10 mg orally daily for generalized anxiety disorder.
Propranolol (Inderal): 20 mg orally every 12 hours as needed for palpitations.

Vital Signs:

Blood Pressure: 140/90 mmHg
Heart Rate: 110 bpm
Respiratory Rate: 20 breaths per minute
Temperature: 98.6°F (37°C)
Oxygen Saturation: 98% on room air

Lab Values:

Complete Blood Count (CBC):
WBC: 8,000/mm³
Hemoglobin: 13.5 g/dL
Platelets: 250,000/mm³
Basic Metabolic Panel (BMP):
Sodium: 138 mEq/L
Potassium: 4.2 mEq/L
Blood Urea Nitrogen (BUN): 18 mg/dL
Creatinine: 0.9 mg/dL
Glucose: 110 mg/dL

Que 1: Considering Mr. Vimal's symptoms and medical history, which medication is most likely contributing to his rapid speech and restlessness?

A) Alprazolam (Xanax)
B) Escitalopram (Lexapro)
C) Propranolol (Inderal)

D) None of the above

Explanation:

Ans 1: The correct answer is B) Escitalopram (Lexapro).

Explanation of Options:

Given Mr. Vimal's symptoms of rapid speech and restlessness, the most likely medication contributing to these side effects is B) Escitalopram (Lexapro). Escitalopram, an SSRI antidepressant, can sometimes cause agitation, restlessness, and other similar symptoms, especially when starting the medication or adjusting the dose1

Que 2: Which of the following statements made by Mr. Vimal describe the effects of his medications on his symptoms?

Options:
A) Mr. Vimal experiences improved heart rate control with Propranolol (Inderal).
B) Mr. Vimal notices increased sedation with Alprazolam (Xanax).
C) Mr. Vimal reports enhanced cognitive function with Alprazolam (Xanax).
D) Mr. Vimal experiences reduced anxiety with Escitalopram (Lexapro).
E) Mr. Vimal reports weight gain as a side effect of Propranolol (Inderal).
F) Mr. Vimal observes improved energy levels with Escitalopram (Lexapro).
G) Mr. Vimal experiences gastrointestinal discomfort with Propranolol (Inderal).
H) Mr. Vimal reports better sleep quality with Alprazolam (Xanax).

Answer:
A) Mr. Vimal experiences improved heart rate control with Propranolol (Inderal).
- **Analysis:** Propranolol is a beta-blocker that reduces heart rate by blocking the effects of adrenaline on beta-adrenergic receptors. This is a well-documented effect of the medication.
- **Correctness: True.**

B) Mr. Vimal notices increased sedation with Alprazolam (Xanax).
- **Analysis:** Alprazolam is a benzodiazepine that enhances GABA activity in the brain, leading to sedation and relaxation. Increased sedation is a common and expected effect of alprazolam.
- **Correctness: True.**

C) Mr. Vimal reports enhanced cognitive function with Alprazolam (Xanax).
- **Analysis:** Alprazolam can cause cognitive impairment, including confusion, memory problems, and reduced concentration. Enhanced cognitive function is not a typical effect of this medication.
- **Correctness: False.**

D) Mr. Vimal experiences reduced anxiety with Escitalopram (Lexapro).
- **Analysis:** Escitalopram is an SSRI commonly prescribed for anxiety disorders. It works by increasing serotonin levels in the brain, which helps reduce anxiety over time. This is a correct statement if Mr. Vimal has been on the medication long enough for it to take effect.
- **Correctness: True.**

E) Mr. Vimal reports weight gain as a side effect of Propranolol (Inderal).
- **Analysis:** Weight gain is a known but less common side effect of propranolol due to its metabolic effects and potential reduction in physical activity caused by fatigue. This statement could be accurate for some patients.
- **Correctness: True.**

F) Mr. Vimal observes improved energy levels with Escitalopram (Lexapro).
- **Analysis:** Escitalopram can initially cause fatigue or drowsiness, especially during the first few weeks of treatment. Improved energy levels are more likely to occur after the medication has taken full effect (4–6 weeks), but this is not a universal experience.
- **Correctness: False.** (This is less likely to be a consistent or immediate effect.)

G) Mr. Vimal experiences gastrointestinal discomfort with Propranolol (Inderal).
- **Analysis:** Gastrointestinal discomfort is not a common side effect of propranolol. More frequent side effects include fatigue, bradycardia, and cold extremities. This statement is unlikely to be accurate.
- **Correctness: False.**

H) Mr. Vimal reports better sleep quality with Alprazolam (Xanax).
- **Analysis:** Alprazolam has sedative properties and can improve sleep quality by reducing anxiety and promoting relaxation. This is a plausible effect of the medication.
- **Correctness: True.**

Que 3 : In the nursing management of Mr. Vimal's anxiety, which of the following actions would be appropriate?

Options:

A) Administering a higher dose of Alprazolam (Xanax) to quickly alleviate his symptoms.
B) Encouraging Mr. Vimal to engage in deep-breathing exercises to help manage anxiety.
C) Advising Mr. Vimal to stop taking Escitalopram (Lexapro) immediately.
D) Suggesting that Mr. Vimal discontinue Propranolol (Inderal) to reduce restlessness.
E) Recommending an increase in the frequency of Alprazolam (Xanax) intake for better anxiety control.
F) Initiating a referral to a mental health professional for counseling and support.
G) Instructing Mr. Vimal to avoid any form of physical activity to minimize stress.

Ans 3:

Explanation:

The correct actions are B) Encouraging Mr. Vimal to engage in deep-breathing exercises to help manage anxiety and F) Initiating a referral to a mental health professional for counseling and support.

Explanation of Options:

A) Incorrect. Administering a higher dose of Alprazolam may not be appropriate and could lead to unwanted side effects.
B) Correct. Deep-breathing exercises are a non-pharmacological intervention to help manage anxiety.
C) Incorrect. Abruptly stopping Escitalopram (Lexapro) can lead to withdrawal symptoms, and any changes should be discussed with the healthcare provider.

D) Incorrect. Discontinuing Propranolol (Inderal) may not be advisable without consulting the healthcare provider, as it is prescribed for palpitations.
E) Incorrect. Increasing the frequency of Alprazolam (Xanax) intake without medical guidance can pose risks of dependence and side effects.
F) Correct. Referring Mr. Vimal to a mental health professional is appropriate for counseling and additional support.
G) Incorrect. Physical activity can be beneficial for managing stress, and avoiding it entirely is not recommended.

Que 4: Regarding the use of antianxiety medications, which statements are correct?

Options:

A) Alprazolam (Xanax) is a selective serotonin reuptake inhibitor (SSRI).
B) Escitalopram (Lexapro) is a benzodiazepine.
C) Propranolol (Inderal) primarily acts on the central nervous system to reduce anxiety.
D) Alprazolam (Xanax) should be abruptly stopped if side effects occur.
E) Escitalopram (Lexapro) may take several weeks to show its full therapeutic effect.
F) Propranolol (Inderal) is contraindicated in individuals with a history of palpitations.
G) Alprazolam (Xanax) may cause drowsiness and impair cognitive function.
H) Escitalopram (Lexapro) is commonly prescribed for immediate relief of acute anxiety.

Ans 4:
Explanation:

The correct statements are E) Escitalopram (Lexapro) may take several weeks to show its full therapeutic effect, G) Alprazolam (Xanax) may cause drowsiness and impair cognitive function

Explanation of Options:

A) Incorrect. Alprazolam (Xanax) is a benzodiazepine, not an SSRI.
B) Incorrect. Escitalopram (Lexapro) is an SSRI, not a benzodiazepine.
C) Incorrect. Propranolol is a beta-blocker that primarily acts on the peripheral nervous system by blocking the effects of adrenaline on beta-adrenergic receptors. It reduces physical symptoms of anxiety (e.g., palpitations, tremors) but does not directly affect the central nervous system.
D) Incorrect. Abruptly stopping Alprazolam (Xanax) can lead to withdrawal symptoms, and any changes should be discussed with the healthcare provider.
E) Correct. Escitalopram (Lexapro) often requires several weeks of use to achieve its full therapeutic effect.
F) Incorrect. Propranolol (Inderal) is prescribed for palpitations, and it is not contraindicated in individuals with a history of palpitations.
G) Correct. Alprazolam (Xanax) can cause drowsiness and impair cognitive function, especially when first starting the medication.
H) Incorrect. Escitalopram (Lexapro) is not commonly prescribed for immediate relief of acute anxiety; its therapeutic effect usually takes time to develop.

Que 5: Which of the following physiological parameters is most likely to be affected by chronic stress?

A) Increased heart rate
B) Elevated platelet count
C) Decreased blood pressure
D) Reduced respiratory rate

Ans 5:
A) Increased heart rate

Explanation:
Chronic stress activates the body's stress response, leading to the release of stress hormones such as adrenaline and cortisol. These hormones can cause various physiological changes, including an increased heart rate. Over time, chronic stress can also contribute to other cardiovascular issues such as high blood pressure and increased risk of heart disease.

Que 6: Read the following nurse's advice

Mr. Vimal, it's essential to address your anxiety symptoms effectively. Firstly, continue taking your prescribed medications as directed by your healthcare provider. Ensure that you are taking Alprazolam (Xanax) as needed for anxiety relief, Escitalopram (Lexapro) for your generalized anxiety disorder, and Propranolol (Inderal) as needed for palpitations. Secondly, consider incorporating relaxation techniques into your daily routine. Deep-breathing exercises and mindfulness can help alleviate stress. Additionally, maintaining a consistent sleep schedule is crucial for overall well-being, so aim for 7-9 hours of quality sleep each night. Moreover, try to identify and address specific stressors in your work environment, seeking support or making changes where possible. Regular physical activity is beneficial for both mental and physical health, so engage in activities you enjoy. Remember to stay hydrated and maintain a balanced diet to support your overall health. Lastly, if you notice any unusual side effects or worsening symptoms, promptly consult your healthcare provider for further guidance.

Identify 2 Incorrect Sentences !

Ans 6:

"Ensure that you are taking Alprazolam (Xanax) as needed for anxiety relief, Escitalopram (Lexapro) for your generalized anxiety disorder, and Propranolol (Inderal) as needed for palpitations."

Explanation:

Incorrect. This sentence suggests that Mr. Vimal should take Propranolol (Inderal) as needed for palpitations, which may not be appropriate. Propranolol is typically prescribed regularly for preventive management of palpitations.

Case Study 16: Management of Geriatric Patients

1. History and Nurse Notes:

Mrs. Margaret Thompson, an 80-year-old female, is admitted to the medical-surgical unit with complaints of generalized weakness, shortness of breath, and confusion. She has a medical history of hypertension, type 2 diabetes, and osteoarthritis. The patient lives alone, and her daughter brought her to the hospital.

Nurse Notes:

Upon admission, Mrs. Thompson appeared fatigued and disoriented.
Blood pressure: 160/90 mmHg, Heart rate: 98 bpm, Respiratory rate: 22 bpm, Temperature: 99.2°F.
Mrs. Thompson has difficulty recalling recent events, and her daughter reports a decline in overall cognitive function over the past few weeks.
The patient complains of joint pain and stiffness in her knees.
Medication reconciliation reveals she is taking metformin, lisinopril, and ibuprofen for arthritis.

2. Medications:

a) Metformin (Glucophage):

Purpose: To manage type 2 diabetes.
Dosage: 1000 mg orally twice a day.
Side effects: GI upset, lactic acidosis (rare).

b) Lisinopril (Prinivil):

Purpose: To control hypertension.
Dosage: 10 mg orally once daily.
Side effects: Cough, hypotension.

c) Ibuprofen (Advil):

Purpose: To alleviate arthritis pain.
Dosage: 200 mg orally every 6 hours as needed.
Side effects: GI bleeding, renal impairment.

3. Vital Signs:

Blood Pressure: 150/85 mmHg
Heart Rate: 92 bpm
Respiratory Rate: 20 bpm
Temperature: 98.8°F
Oxygen Saturation: 95%

4. Lab Reports:
Fasting glucose: 160 mg/dL (elevated).
HbA1c: 8.5% (poorly controlled diabetes).
Blood Urea Nitrogen (BUN): 28 mg/dL (elevated).
Serum Creatinine: 1.5 mg/dL (elevated).
C-reactive protein (CRP): 15 mg/L (elevated).

Que 1: What is a potential concern in managing pain for older adults with arthritis, especially those with hypertension?

a) Increased risk of cognitive decline

b) Adverse effects on renal function

c) Improved cardiovascular health

d) Enhanced joint mobility

Ans 1:

Explanation:
Correct Answer: b) Adverse effects on renal function

Arthritis pain management often involves nonsteroidal anti-inflammatory drugs (NSAIDs), which may pose a risk to renal function, especially in older adults with hypertension. NSAIDs can lead to fluid retention and increased blood pressure, potentially exacerbating hypertension and causing renal impairment.
Incorrect Options:
a) Increased risk of cognitive decline

While chronic pain may impact cognitive function, the primary concern with arthritis pain management in this case is related to renal function due to the use of NSAIDs.
c) Improved cardiovascular health

Pain management strategies may impact cardiovascular health indirectly, but the primary focus is on potential adverse effects on renal function, not cardiovascular improvement.
d) Enhanced joint mobility

While the goal of arthritis management is to improve joint mobility, the question specifically addresses concerns related to hypertension and pain management. The use of NSAIDs and their potential impact on renal function is the primary concern in this context.

Que 2: What considerations should be taken into account when managing medications for an elderly patient with multiple chronic conditions?

a) Prioritize pain management over blood pressure control

b) Adjust dosages without considering potential drug interactions

c) Monitor renal function due to potential adverse effects

d) Focus solely on cardiovascular health

e) Overlook potential side effects of medications

f) Assume that cognitive decline is unrelated to medication management

g) Neglect regular vital sign monitoring

h) Disregard the impact of medication on joint mobility

Ans 2:

c) Monitor renal function due to potential adverse effects

- It's crucial to monitor renal function because many medications can have adverse effects on the kidneys, especially in elderly patients.

Other Considerations:
- **Avoid** prioritizing pain management over blood pressure control (a): Both pain management and blood pressure control are important and should be balanced.
- **Avoid** adjusting dosages without considering potential drug interactions (b): Always consider drug interactions to prevent adverse effects.
- **Avoid** focusing solely on cardiovascular health (d): Comprehensive care should address all health concerns, not just cardiovascular health.
- **Avoid** overlooking potential side effects of medications (e): Be vigilant about potential side effects to ensure patient safety.
- **Avoid** assuming cognitive decline is unrelated to medication management (f): Medications can impact cognitive function, and this should be considered.
- **Avoid** neglecting regular vital sign monitoring (g): Regular monitoring of vital signs is essential for managing overall health.
- **Avoid** disregarding the impact of medication on joint mobility (h): Consider how medications may affect joint mobility and overall physical function.

Que 3: Which of the following statements made by the nurse indicates she needs training on providing care for an elderly patient with arthritis and hypertension?

a) "I'll prioritize blood pressure control over addressing the patient's joint pain."

b) "Arthritis medications won't affect the patient's renal function."

c) "Regular monitoring of vital signs isn't necessary for elderly patients with chronic conditions."

d) "I'll adjust medication dosages without considering potential drug interactions."

e) "Cognitive decline is unrelated to the medications prescribed for arthritis."

f) "Joint mobility is not a significant concern in managing arthritis in the elderly."

g) "I won't consider potential side effects; the patient can report if something feels wrong."

Ans 3: Statements indicating the need for training: b, c, d, e, f, g

b) "Arthritis medications won't affect the patient's renal function."
- **Explanation:** Arthritis medications, such as NSAIDs, can adversely affect renal function, especially in elderly patients with hypertension. Monitoring renal function is crucial.

c) "Regular monitoring of vital signs isn't necessary for elderly patients with chronic conditions."
- **Explanation:** Regular monitoring of vital signs is essential for managing chronic conditions in elderly patients to detect and address any potential issues promptly.

d) "I'll adjust medication dosages without considering potential drug interactions."
   - **Explanation:** Considering potential drug interactions is crucial when adjusting medication dosages to prevent adverse effects and ensure patient safety.

e) **"Cognitive decline is unrelated to the medications prescribed for arthritis."**
   - **Explanation:** Some medications can affect cognitive function, especially in elderly patients. It is important to consider the potential impact of medications on cognitive health.

f) **"Joint mobility is not a significant concern in managing arthritis in the elderly."**
   - **Explanation:** Joint mobility is a significant concern in managing arthritis. Maintaining and improving joint mobility is essential for overall well-being and quality of life in elderly patients.

g) **"I won't consider potential side effects; the patient can report if something feels wrong."**
   - **Explanation:** Actively monitoring for potential side effects is crucial to ensure patient safety and to address any adverse effects promptly.

Que 4: Fill in the Blank Choice Question:

The patient with a history of hypertension and arthritis, is prescribed _____ to manage joint pain. Considering his hypertension, it is crucial to monitor _____ and adjust medications to prevent adverse effects on renal function.

Options:

a) Ibuprofen, blood glucose levels

b) Acetaminophen, respiratory rate

c) Naproxen, renal function

Ans 4:
Explanation:

Correct Answer: c) Naproxen, renal function

The patient experiencing joint pain due to arthritis, may be prescribed NSAIDs such as naproxen for pain management. Considering his hypertension, monitoring renal function is crucial due to the potential adverse effects of NSAIDs on the kidneys.
Incorrect Options:

a) Ibuprofen, blood glucose levels

While ibuprofen is an NSAID commonly used for pain, monitoring blood glucose levels is not directly related to its use. Renal function is more relevant in this context.
b) Acetaminophen, respiratory rate

Acetaminophen is not an NSAID and is less likely to affect renal function. Respiratory rate monitoring is not directly related to arthritis medication.
This question assesses the understanding of appropriate arthritis medication choices and the importance of monitoring specific parameters, especially in the context of hypertension.

Que 5: Fill in the Blank Choice Question:

When managing an elderly patient with arthritis, it is essential to assess _____ as these medications may impact renal function. Additionally, regular monitoring of _____ is crucial, especially considering the patient's history of hypertension.

Options:

a) Cognitive function, blood pressure

b) Joint mobility, blood glucose levels

c) Renal function, vital signs

Ans 5:
Explanation:

Correct Answer: c) Renal function, vital signs

Arthritis medications, especially NSAIDs, can potentially impact renal function. Monitoring renal function is crucial to prevent adverse effects. Additionally, regular vital sign monitoring, including blood pressure, is essential, especially in patients with a history of hypertension.
Incorrect Options:

a) Cognitive function, blood pressure

While cognitive function is important, the primary concern related to arthritis medications in this case is renal function. Blood pressure monitoring is also crucial but not directly related to arthritis medications.
b) Joint mobility, blood glucose levels

Joint mobility is a concern in arthritis management, but the question emphasizes the impact of medications on renal function. Blood glucose levels are not directly related to arthritis medications.
This question evaluates knowledge related to monitoring parameters when managing arthritis medications in an elderly patient with hypertension.

Que 6: Which of the following side effects should the nurse be particularly vigilant for in this case? (Select two options)

a) Gastrointestinal bleeding

b) Increased blood glucose levels

c) Renal impairment

d) Cough

e) Cognitive decline

f) Enhanced joint mobility

Ans 6:
Explanation:

Correct Answers: a) Gastrointestinal bleeding and c) Renal impairment

Gastrointestinal bleeding (a): NSAIDs, commonly prescribed for arthritis, can increase the risk of gastrointestinal bleeding. Monitoring for symptoms such as black stools or abdominal pain is crucial.

Renal impairment (c): NSAIDs, including those used for arthritis, may impact renal function. Regular monitoring of renal function is essential to detect any signs of impairment, such as changes in BUN and serum creatinine levels.

Incorrect Options:

b) Increased blood glucose levels

Arthritis medications, particularly NSAIDs, are not known to significantly affect blood glucose levels. This side effect is less relevant in this context.

d) Cough

Cough is a potential side effect of medications like ACE inhibitors, commonly used for hypertension. However, it is not directly related to arthritis medications in this case.

e) Cognitive decline

While cognitive decline may be a concern in elderly patients, it is not a common side effect of arthritis medications. This option is less relevant in the context of Mr. Johnson's case.

f) Enhanced joint mobility

Enhanced joint mobility is a desired outcome of arthritis management. It is not a side effect but a positive effect of appropriate treatment. This option is incorrect in the context of potential side effects.

CASE STUDY 17: Infection Control in a Postoperative Patient

Patient History and Nurse's Notes:
Mrs. Martha Rodriguez, a 55-year-old female, underwent abdominal surgery for appendicitis three days ago. She has a history of type 2 diabetes managed with oral hypoglycemic agents. Mrs. Rodriguez is currently admitted to the surgical unit for postoperative care.

Nurse's Notes:

Postoperative recovery has been progressing as expected, with controlled pain and stable vital signs. Mrs. Rodriguez complains of mild incisional pain but denies any signs of infection such as increased redness, swelling, or discharge.
Regular glucose monitoring reveals well-controlled blood sugar levels.
The surgical wound appears clean and dry, with intact staples in place.

Medications:
a) Ceftriaxone (Rocephin):

Purpose: Prophylactic antibiotic to prevent surgical site infection.
Dosage: 1g IV every 24 hours.
Duration: 48 hours postoperatively.
b) Acetaminophen (Tylenol):

Purpose: Pain management.
Dosage: 650mg orally every 4-6 hours as needed.

Vital Signs:

Blood Pressure: 120/80 mmHg (Normal range: 90/60 to 120/80 mmHg)
Heart Rate: 80 bpm (Normal range: 60 to 100 bpm)
Respiratory Rate: 18 bpm (Normal range: 12 to 20 bpm)
Temperature: 98.6°F (Normal range: 97.8 to 99.1°F)
Oxygen Saturation: 98% (Normal range: 95% to 100%)

Lab Reports:

Lab Reports:
a) White Blood Cell (WBC) Count:

Within normal range (Normal range: 4,000 to 11,000 cells/mcL).
b) Blood Glucose Level:

Within target range for a patient with diabetes (Normal range: 70 to 130 mg/dL).
c) C-reactive Protein (CRP):

Normal range, indicating no significant inflammation (Normal range: 0 to 1 mg/dL).

Que 1: Which aspect of Mrs. Rodriguez's postoperative status indicates successful infection control?

A) Increased redness around the surgical wound.

B) Complaints of severe incisional pain.

C) Stable vital signs and well-controlled blood sugar levels.

D) Discharge from the surgical wound.

E) Presence of intact staples.

Ans 1:

Explanation:

A) Increased redness around the surgical wound (Incorrect):

Redness is a sign of inflammation, which could indicate infection. Mrs. Rodriguez denies signs of infection, and the wound appears clean and dry, making increased redness unlikely.
B) Complaints of severe incisional pain (Incorrect):

Severe pain may indicate a problem, but Mrs. Rodriguez complains of mild incisional pain. Pain alone is not a reliable indicator of infection in this case.
C) Stable vital signs and well-controlled blood sugar levels (Correct):

Stable vital signs (blood pressure, heart rate, respiratory rate, temperature, and oxygen saturation) and well-controlled blood sugar levels indicate a favorable postoperative recovery without signs of infection.
D) Discharge from the surgical wound (Incorrect):

Discharge is a sign of infection, and Mrs. Rodriguez denies any signs of infection. The wound appears clean and dry, making the presence of discharge unlikely.
E) Presence of intact staples (Incorrect):

While intact staples are a positive sign, they alone do not confirm infection control. The overall assessment, including vital signs and absence of signs of infection, is more indicative of successful infection control.

Que 2: Which of the following statements by the nurse needs correction in the management and care of Mrs. Rodriguez, a postoperative patient?

A) "Administering Ceftriaxone for 48 hours postoperatively helps prevent surgical site infection."

B) "Acetaminophen is prescribed every 2 hours for effective pain management."

C) "Monitoring Mrs. Rodriguez's blood pressure, heart rate, and respiratory rate every 4 hours is sufficient."

D) "Pain assessment should include asking about the location, intensity, and quality of pain."

E) "Regular glucose monitoring is essential to ensure well-controlled blood sugar levels."

F) "The presence of mild incisional pain is expected during the early postoperative period."

G) "Inspecting the surgical wound for signs of infection is part of routine nursing care."

H) "Administering Ceftriaxone beyond 48 hours postoperatively enhances its prophylactic effects."

Ans 2:

Explanation:

A) "Administering Ceftriaxone for 48 hours postoperatively helps prevent surgical site infection." (Correct):

This statement is correct. Prophylactic antibiotics, like Ceftriaxone, are often prescribed for a specific duration postoperatively to prevent surgical site infections.
B) "Acetaminophen is prescribed every 2 hours for effective pain management." (Incorrect):

Acetaminophen is usually prescribed every 4-6 hours, not every 2 hours. This statement needs correction to avoid potential medication errors.
C) "Monitoring Mrs. Rodriguez's blood pressure, heart rate, and respiratory rate every 4 hours is sufficient." (Incorrect):

Monitoring vital signs every 4 hours may not be frequent enough during the early postoperative period. Continuous or more frequent monitoring may be necessary for early detection of any complications.
D) "Pain assessment should include asking about the location, intensity, and quality of pain." (Correct):

This statement is correct. Comprehensive pain assessment includes gathering information about the location, intensity, and quality of pain.
E) "Regular glucose monitoring is essential to ensure well-controlled blood sugar levels." (Correct):

This statement is correct. Regular glucose monitoring is crucial for patients with diabetes to maintain well-controlled blood sugar levels.
F) "The presence of mild incisional pain is expected during the early postoperative period." (Correct):

This statement is correct. Mild incisional pain is common in the early postoperative period, and it aligns with the expected recovery process.
G) "Inspecting the surgical wound for signs of infection is part of routine nursing care." (Correct):

This statement is correct. Routine inspection of the surgical wound is essential for early detection of any signs of infection.
H) "Administering Ceftriaxone beyond 48 hours postoperatively enhances its prophylactic effects." (Incorrect):

Continuing prophylactic antibiotics beyond the recommended duration may not necessarily enhance their effects and may contribute to antibiotic resistance. This statement needs correction.
In summary, the correct answers are B ("Acetaminophen is prescribed every 2 hours for effective pain management.") and C ("Monitoring Mrs. Rodriguez's blood pressure, heart rate, and respiratory rate every 4 hours is sufficient."), as these statements require correction in the context of nursing management and care of postoperative patients.

Que 3: Mrs. Rodriguez's blood glucose level is within the target range for a patient with diabetes, ranging from ____ to ____ mg/dL. This indicates that her diabetes is _____ controlled.

Options:

A) 50 to 150; moderately

B) 70 to 130; well

C) 90 to 180; poorly

D) 60 to 120; adequately

Ans 3: Explanation:

A) 50 to 150; moderately (Incorrect):

The correct blood glucose range for a patient with diabetes is not 50 to 150 mg/dL. This option provides an incorrect range and suggests moderate control, which is not supported by the case study.
B) 70 to 130; well (Correct):

The target range for blood glucose levels in a patient with diabetes is generally 70 to 130 mg/dL. This option provides the correct range, and the term "well" indicates that her diabetes is well-controlled, aligning with the information in the case study.
C) 90 to 180; poorly (Incorrect):

The correct blood glucose range is not 90 to 180 mg/dL. This option provides an incorrect range, and the term "poorly" suggests poor control, which is not supported by the case study.
D) 60 to 120; adequately (Incorrect):

The correct blood glucose range is not 60 to 120 mg/dL. This option provides an incorrect range, and the term "adequately" does not accurately describe the well-controlled blood glucose levels mentioned in the case study.

Que 4: Mrs. Rodriguez is prescribed Ceftriaxone, a prophylactic antibiotic, for ____ hours postoperatively to prevent surgical site infection. This antibiotic is administered at a dosage of ____ IV every 24 hours.

Options:

A) 24; 500mg

B) 48; 1g

C) 72; 750mg

D) 36; 2g

Ans 4:

Explanation:

A) 24; 500mg (Incorrect):

This option provides an incorrect duration and dosage for the administration of Ceftriaxone. The correct duration mentioned in the case study is longer, and the correct dosage is higher.

B) 48; 1g (Correct):

The case study mentions that Ceftriaxone is prescribed for 48 hours postoperatively at a dosage of 1g IV every 24 hours. This option accurately reflects the information provided.

C) 72; 750mg (Incorrect):

This option provides an incorrect duration and dosage for the administration of Ceftriaxone. The correct duration mentioned in the case study is shorter, and the correct dosage is lower.

D) 36; 2g (Incorrect):

This option provides an incorrect duration and dosage for the administration of Ceftriaxone. The correct duration mentioned in the case study is longer, and the correct dosage is lower.

Que 5: Which vital sign is particularly crucial to monitor for Mrs. Rodriguez, given her history of type 2 diabetes, during the postoperative period?

A) Respiratory rate

B) Blood pressure

C) Heart rate

D) Temperature

E) Oxygen saturation

Ans 5: D) Temperature
Explanation:
- Monitoring temperature is essential for identifying potential infections, especially in postoperative patients with diabetes. People with diabetes are at a higher risk of infections, and elevated temperature can be an early sign of infection or sepsis, which requires prompt medical attention.

Que 6: Which intervention is most effective for infection control in postoperative patients like Mrs. Rodriguez?

A) Administering pain medication regularly

B) Keeping the surgical wound moist for faster healing

C) Using strict aseptic techniques during wound care

D) Encouraging early ambulation for improved blood circulation

Explanation:

A) Administering pain medication regularly (Incorrect):

While pain management is important for postoperative patients, it is not a direct intervention for infection control. Infection control focuses on preventing and managing infections, and pain medication does not address this aspect.

B) Keeping the surgical wound moist for faster healing (Incorrect):

Keeping the surgical wound moist may contribute to wound healing, but it does not directly address infection control. In fact, excessive moisture can potentially create a breeding ground for bacteria, highlighting the importance of proper wound care.

C) Using strict aseptic techniques during wound care (Correct):

Strict aseptic techniques during wound care, such as using sterile instruments and maintaining a sterile field, are essential for infection control. This helps prevent the introduction of pathogens into the surgical site and reduces the risk of postoperative infections.

D) Encouraging early ambulation for improved blood circulation (Incorrect):

Early ambulation is beneficial for various aspects of postoperative recovery, including blood circulation, but it is not a direct intervention for infection control. Infection control measures focus on preventing and minimizing the risk of infections in postoperative patients.

CASE STUDY 18 : Nutrition and Medication Interaction

Patient History:
Mrs. Sarah Thompson, a 62-year-old female, was admitted to the surgical unit for postoperative care following a cholecystectomy (gallbladder removal) due to gallstones. She has a medical history of hypertension and is currently prescribed Lisinopril, an angiotensin-converting enzyme (ACE) inhibitor, to manage her blood pressure.

Nursing Notes:
Postoperative recovery has been progressing well for Mrs. Thompson. She reports minimal incisional pain, and her vital signs remain stable. The surgical wound is clean and dry, with no signs of infection. Mrs. Thompson is ambulating independently and adhering to the prescribed diet.

Medications:
a) Lisinopril (Zestril):

Purpose: Management of hypertension.
Dosage: 10mg orally once daily.
b) Acetaminophen (Tylenol):

Purpose: Pain management.
Dosage: 500mg orally every 4-6 hours as needed for pain.

Lab Values:
a) Serum Creatinine: 0.9 mg/dL (Normal range: 0.6 to 1.2 mg/dL)
b) Blood Glucose Level: 110 mg/dL (Normal range: 70 to 130 mg/dL)
c) Hemoglobin A1c: 6.2% (Normal range: Less than 5.7%)

Vital Signs:

Blood Pressure: 128/78 mmHg (Normal range: Less than 120/80 mmHg)
Heart Rate: 72 bpm (Normal range: 60 to 100 bpm)
Respiratory Rate: 18 bpm (Normal range: 12 to 20 bpm)
Temperature: 98.4°F (Normal range: 97.8 to 99.1°F)
Oxygen Saturation: 97% (Normal range: 95% to 100%)

Que 1: Considering the postoperative care of Mrs. Sarah Thompson, who underwent a cholecystectomy, which statement about Total Parenteral Nutrition (TPN) is accurate?

a) TPN is typically indicated for patients with normal gastrointestinal function.

b) TPN may be considered if enteral nutrition is contraindicated or insufficient.

c) TPN is a primary source of postoperative pain management.

d) TPN administration can be initiated without monitoring serum electrolyte levels.

e) TPN is mainly prescribed for patients with a high oral intake of nutrients.

Ans 1:
Explanation:

a) Incorrect. TPN is usually reserved for patients with compromised or impaired gastrointestinal function, such as those who cannot tolerate enteral nutrition.

b) Correct. TPN may be considered when enteral nutrition (feeding through the gastrointestinal tract) is contraindicated or insufficient. In certain cases, such as bowel obstruction or severe malabsorption, TPN becomes necessary.

c) Incorrect. TPN is not used for pain management. It is a form of intravenous nutrition that provides essential nutrients but does not address pain relief.

d) Incorrect. TPN administration requires careful monitoring of serum electrolyte levels, as imbalances can occur. Regular assessments are crucial to prevent complications.

e) Incorrect. TPN is not typically prescribed for patients with a high oral intake of nutrients. It is reserved for situations where oral or enteral intake is not feasible or sufficient.

Que 2:
Which of the following considerations should be taken into account when managing Mrs. Sarah Thompson's postoperative care, considering her medical history and medications? Select the two correct options.

a) Increasing the dosage of Lisinopril for better blood pressure control.

b) Monitoring Mrs. Thompson's blood glucose levels closely.

c) Administering Ibuprofen for pain management.

d) Assessing serum creatinine levels regularly.

e) Adding a calcium supplement to Mrs. Thompson's medication regimen.

f) Encouraging Mrs. Thompson to limit ambulation to prevent postoperative complications.

g) Discontinuing Lisinopril temporarily to avoid interactions with pain medications.

Ans 2:
Explanation:

a) Incorrect. Increasing the dosage of Lisinopril without specific indications may lead to hypotension, especially in the postoperative period.

b) Correct. Mrs. Thompson's medical history includes hypertension, and Lisinopril, her prescribed medication, may impact blood glucose levels. Monitoring blood glucose is crucial to ensure proper management.

c) Incorrect. Ibuprofen is not recommended due to its potential impact on bleeding risk postoperatively. Acetaminophen is the preferred pain management option in this case.

d) Correct. Monitoring serum creatinine levels is essential, especially considering Mrs. Thompson's use of Lisinopril, which can affect renal function.

e) Incorrect. There is no indication or evidence in the case study to support the addition of a calcium supplement to Mrs. Thompson's medication regimen.

f) Incorrect. Encouraging ambulation is appropriate for postoperative care, and limiting ambulation may lead to complications.

g) Incorrect. Discontinuing Lisinopril abruptly can have adverse effects on blood pressure control, and it is not recommended without proper medical supervision.

Que 3: Mrs. Sarah Thompson, a 62-year-old female, underwent a cholecystectomy and is currently prescribed _____ (a) for blood pressure management and _____ (b) for pain relief. It is crucial to monitor her _____ (c) levels due to potential interactions with the medications.

Options:

a) Ibuprofen

b) Acetaminophen

c) Serum Creatinine

d) Lisinopril

Ans 3:
Explanation:

a) Incorrect. Mrs. Thompson is prescribed Lisinopril for blood pressure management, not Ibuprofen. Ibuprofen is not recommended due to its potential impact on bleeding risk postoperatively.

b) Correct. Mrs. Thompson is prescribed Acetaminophen for pain relief after her cholecystectomy. It is the appropriate medication for postoperative pain management.

c) Correct. Monitoring serum creatinine levels is essential, especially considering Mrs. Thompson's use of Lisinopril, an angiotensin-converting enzyme (ACE) inhibitor. Lisinopril can affect renal function, and regular monitoring is crucial to identify any adverse effects.

Que 4: Which of the following statements by the nurse needs consideration for the correct administration of Total Parenteral Nutrition (TPN) in postoperative care? Select the two correct options.

a) "TPN should be infused rapidly to ensure a quick delivery of nutrients."

b) "Regularly assessing the patient's blood glucose levels is unnecessary during TPN."

c) "Changing the TPN solution and tubing every 24 hours is a standard practice to prevent infection."

d) "Adding medications to the TPN bag is recommended for efficient administration."

e) "Monitoring for signs of complications, such as infection or hyperglycemia, is essential."

f) "TPN is the first-line choice for patients with intact gastrointestinal function."

g) "Administering TPN through a dedicated central line is preferred over a peripheral line."

h) "Adjusting the TPN rate based on the patient's clinical condition is unnecessary."

Explanation:

a) Incorrect. Rapid infusion of TPN can lead to complications, such as hyperglycemia and electrolyte imbalances. TPN should be administered at a controlled and prescribed rate.

b) Incorrect. Monitoring blood glucose levels is crucial during TPN administration, especially due to the high glucose content in the solution. Regular assessments help prevent hyperglycemia.

c) Correct. Changing the TPN solution and tubing every 24 hours is a standard practice to minimize the risk of infection, ensuring aseptic technique in TPN administration.

d) Incorrect. Adding medications directly to the TPN bag is not recommended as it can lead to compatibility issues and compromise the stability of the solution.

e) Correct. Monitoring for signs of complications, such as infection or hyperglycemia, is essential to ensure patient safety during TPN administration.

f) Incorrect. TPN is typically reserved for patients with impaired or non-functional gastrointestinal tracts, where enteral nutrition is not feasible.

g) Correct. Administering TPN through a dedicated central line is preferred over a peripheral line to reduce the risk of complications such as thrombophlebitis.

h) Incorrect. Adjusting the TPN rate based on the patient's clinical condition is necessary to meet changing nutritional needs and prevent overinfusion or underinfusion.

Que 5: When considering nutrition and caution in certain medications, which of the following statements are correct? Select the two appropriate options.

a) Increasing the dosage of an anticoagulant is advisable for postoperative patients to prevent clot formation.

b) Monitoring blood glucose levels is important when a patient is prescribed corticosteroids.

c) Administering calcium supplements is recommended in combination with iron supplements for better absorption.

d) Ibuprofen is the preferred choice for pain management in patients with a history of gastrointestinal bleeding.

e) Antidepressants may have interactions with certain foods, such as those containing tyramine, requiring dietary restrictions.

f) Abruptly discontinuing antihypertensive medications is safe during the postoperative period.

Ans 5:
Explanation:

a) Incorrect. Increasing the dosage of anticoagulants without specific indications can elevate the risk of bleeding, which is undesirable in postoperative patients.

b) Correct. Corticosteroids, like other medications, may impact blood glucose levels, necessitating monitoring, especially in patients with diabetes.

c) Incorrect. Calcium and iron supplements should not be taken together, as they can interfere with each other's absorption.

d) Incorrect. Ibuprofen, as a nonsteroidal anti-inflammatory drug (NSAID), can increase the risk of gastrointestinal bleeding, and it is not the preferred choice in patients with a history of such bleeding.

e) Correct. Certain antidepressants, particularly monoamine oxidase inhibitors (MAOIs), can interact with tyramine-containing foods, requiring dietary restrictions to prevent adverse effects.

f) Incorrect. Abruptly discontinuing antihypertensive medications can lead to uncontrolled blood pressure, and it is not safe without proper medical supervision.

Que 6: In the context of Total Parenteral Nutrition (TPN) for postoperative patients like Mrs. Sarah Thompson, which statement is true regarding the administration of TPN?

a) TPN is initiated without considering the patient's nutritional requirements.

b) TPN is a suitable choice for patients with functional gastrointestinal tracts.

c) Monitoring for complications, such as infection and hyperglycemia, is unnecessary during TPN.

d) TPN provides both macro and micronutrients to meet the patient's nutritional needs.

e) TPN is primarily used for short-term nutritional support after surgery.

Ans 6:

Explanation:

a) Incorrect. TPN initiation is based on the patient's specific nutritional requirements and is not initiated without consideration.

b) Incorrect. TPN is typically reserved for patients with impaired or non-functional gastrointestinal tracts, where enteral nutrition is not feasible.

c) Incorrect. Monitoring for complications, including infection and hyperglycemia, is crucial during TPN administration to ensure patient safety.

d) Correct. TPN provides both macro and micronutrients, including proteins, fats, carbohydrates, vitamins, and minerals, to meet the patient's comprehensive nutritional needs.

e) Incorrect. TPN is often used for long-term nutritional support in situations where enteral nutrition is not possible or contraindicated.

Further Reading

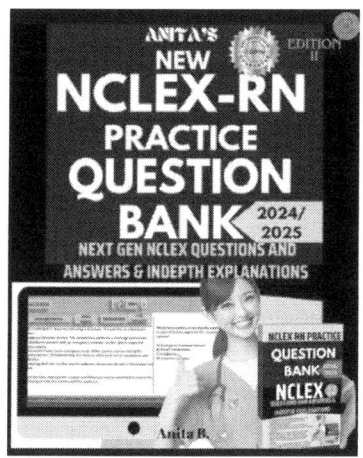

The "**NEW NCLEX RN PRACTICE QUESTION BANK**" is a comprehensive tool designed to help nursing students succeed in the NCLEX exam. Here's a breakdown of its key features:

1. **Extensive Practice**: Contains over 700 well-crafted questions that closely reflect the NCLEX exam's difficulty, helping you prepare with both depth and quality.

2. **Strategic Guidance**: Offers detailed rationales for each question, helping you understand why an answer is correct or incorrect, and provides strategic insights for tackling tricky questions.

3. **Next Generation NCLEX Formats**: Includes practice with new question types like Extended Multiple Response and figure-based questions, ensuring you're prepared for all NCLEX formats.

4. **Enhanced Answer Explanations**: Detailed explanations for answers provide deeper insights, making it easier to understand the reasoning behind each solution.

5. **Question-Solving Strategies**: Features over 400 strategies to effectively approach different types of questions and scenarios.

6. **Clear and Accessible Language**: Uses simplified language to ensure complex medical terms are easy to understand, benefiting students with educational gaps or multiple exam attempts.

7. **Tailored for a Versatile Audience**: Suitable for both new graduates and returning nurses, addressing the unique challenges faced by each group.

8. **Diverse Question Formats**: Covers various NCLEX question types, such as drag-and-drop, prioritization, and ordering questions.

9. **Proven Success**: Trusted by many students who have achieved their nursing goals, serving as an inspiration to others aiming for similar success.

This resource encourages daily practice, strategic preparation, and continuous learning to build the confidence needed to excel on the NCLEX exam. Get it here: **https://a.co/d/7lmJbgY**

Bibliography

Bhattarai, A. (2023). New Next Generation NCLEX RN Question Bank 2023/24: BIGBOOK of Question & Answer Practice (NEW NEXT GENERATION NCLEX RN EXAM INTENSIVE PREPARATION SERIES). Independently published.

Schull, P. (2013). McGraw-Hill Nurses Drug Handbook, Seventh Edition (McGraw-Hill's Nurses Drug Handbook) (7th ed.). McGraw Hill / Medical.

Lippincott Williams & Wilkins. (2021). Nursing2022 Drug Handbook (Nursing Drug Handbook) Forty-Second, North American Edition.

Meloni, S., Medical Creations, & Mastenbjörk, M. (2021). Pharmacology Review - A Comprehensive Reference Guide for Medical, Nursing, and Paramedic Students. Medical Creations.

Bhattarai, A., & Subedi, G. (2023). Mastering New/Next Generation NCLEX RN Pharmacology: Theory, Strategies, and Examples with Case Studies - NEW 2023/24 Guide (NEW ... NCLEX RN EXAM INTENSIVE PREPARATION SERIES). Independently published.

Tucker, R. G. (2021). 2022 Lippincott Pocket Drug Guide for Nurses [Kindle Edition]. Wolters Kluwer Health. ASIN: B09FFNXSYP.

Kaplan Nursing. (2015). NCLEX-RN Drug Guide: 300 Medications You Need to Know for the Exam (Kaplan Test Prep) (Sixth edition). Kaplan Publishing.

Myers, E. (2021). MedSurg Notes: Nurse's Clinical Pocket Guide Fifth Edition (5th ed.). F.A. Davis Company.

THANK YOU !

Dear Reader,

Thank you for taking the time to read 'NCLEX RN CASE STUDIES EXAM PRACTICE BOOTCAMP '. I hope that you found the information and resources in this book helpful as you prepare for the NCLEX exam.

I am grateful for your support and are committed to helping you achieve your goal of becoming a nurse. If you found this book useful, I would greatly appreciate it if you could share it with others who may also benefit from its content.

Please don't hesitate to reach out to me if you have any questions or feedback. I would love to hear from you and hear about your success on the NCLEX exam.

Once again, thank you for choosing NCLEX RN CASE STUDIES EXAM PRACTICE BOOTCAMP and for your continued support of my work.

Sincerely,
Anita Bhattarai